FOR THE GOOD OF ALL

DAVID WILLOCKS

FOR THE GOOD OF ALL

A HANDBOOK FOR HEALING BODY, MIND AND SOUL

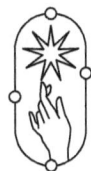

mimosa

First published in 2022 by

mimosa

Istros Books, London, United Kingdom, www.istrosbooks.com

Copyright © David Willocks, 2022

The right of David Willocks, to be identified as the author of this work has been asserted in accordance with the Copyright, Designs and Patents Act, 1988

Compiled and edited by Susan D. Curtis

Photography: David Baird Photography, Christchurch, New Zealand

Typesetting: Davor Pukljak, www.frontispis.hr

ISBN: 978-1-912545-83-4

CONTENTS

A HEALING JOURNEY

New Zealand, 2021-22

In April of 2021, in the middle of the night, I decided that I needed to fly halfway across the world to New Zealand, a place that I had only visited once before, but was nevertheless, my fatherland. The decision came in the midst of a personal crisis that was firmly set in a national and global crisis that had severely disrupted the majority of people's lives. The impulse for understanding and healing were strong within me, although the method and means were not then known to me. I simply decided to follow my intuition and feed my faith, while overcoming my fears.

The preparations for my adventure involved clearing the contents of my central London office and my apartment, which provided a wonderful distraction from the doubts which came at me from all sides. In just over three months, I managed to give away or pack away all my possessions, and had found a tenant for my property: the perfect match of someone who urgently needed a place in London linked through a mutual and trusted friend. Travel involves money of course, as well as logistical preparations, safeguards, etc. My father had provided me with NZ citizenship, my divorce with some spare cash, and my self-run publishing business with the ability to work remotely, as long as I remained efficient and well-prepared. While I flew 11,400 miles in July 2021, there were translators working from Croatian and Slovenian for books I would publish that autumn and the following spring; there was a talented designer waiting in Croatia for any graphic work that needed doing; there were book reps in Newcastle looking after stock and sales.

It took me a while to get accustomed to a new island, then to move to a more southern one, and to then find myself in the place I needed to be; which turned out to be the city of Christchurch and the surrounding region of Canterbury. The names were all too familiar, although the landscape was more rugged, more dramatic and much less populated. It was here that I met David Willocks, a quiet and unassuming man who carries his magic unobtrusively. And I do mean magic, for during the months I spent learning his art while preparing this book, I discovered that dowsing can open the door to one's true self by revealing the wonders which lie around us in nature. This is magic that has always existed and been available to humanity, but which we have been educated and conditioned to ignore or reject. It is the magic of the poet, who knew long before polygraphs that the human heart beats the rhythm of truth. It is the magic of the spirits of the land, the gods of place and the oracles of wisdom that all humans have believed in and respected throughout their history, until we were relatively recently led away from that path.

It may well be time to find our way once again. Science and health – like much of education – have become businesses that operate within a matrix of interests and agendas that are often contrary to the greater good. The energy and healing power of the earth has always been freely available to us, with the only payment required being time, patience and humility.

Some knowledge of esoteric science, as well as a belief in the divine, are assumed in these pages, but are not a requirement. When I arrived in Christchurch and met David, I was on a journey with an unknown destination and no map: as time went on and I began to learn from him, I received confirmation that the corrosive power of bitterness and negativity have detrimental effects on one's health, and that there is a healing power in compassion and forgiveness, when applied to oneself and to others. David takes as a prerequisite that healing is possible and available. He takes for granted the love of God – or the goodness of the universe if you prefer – and he researches and practises his art until he finds the most efficient and beneficial way to help.

It was an open heart and mind that enabled me to start healing, and the tangible existence of this book is a testament to the ever-present power of renewal. Here you will find simple advice about diet and fitness, along with explorations of the more spiritual side of healing involving auras, meridian lines and the chakra system (our personal energy fields), ley lines (the earth's energy fields) and the energetic signatures of all that exists (the vibrational makeup of material and intangible phenomena which we tap into as we dowse). Everything contained in these pages has been composed, explained and published for the good of all. It is the first title of a new imprint that was inspired by and conceived during my time in New Zealand – *mimosa* books, named after the second star of the Southern Cross, a constellation beloved of the peoples of that nation and region.

Susan D. Curtis

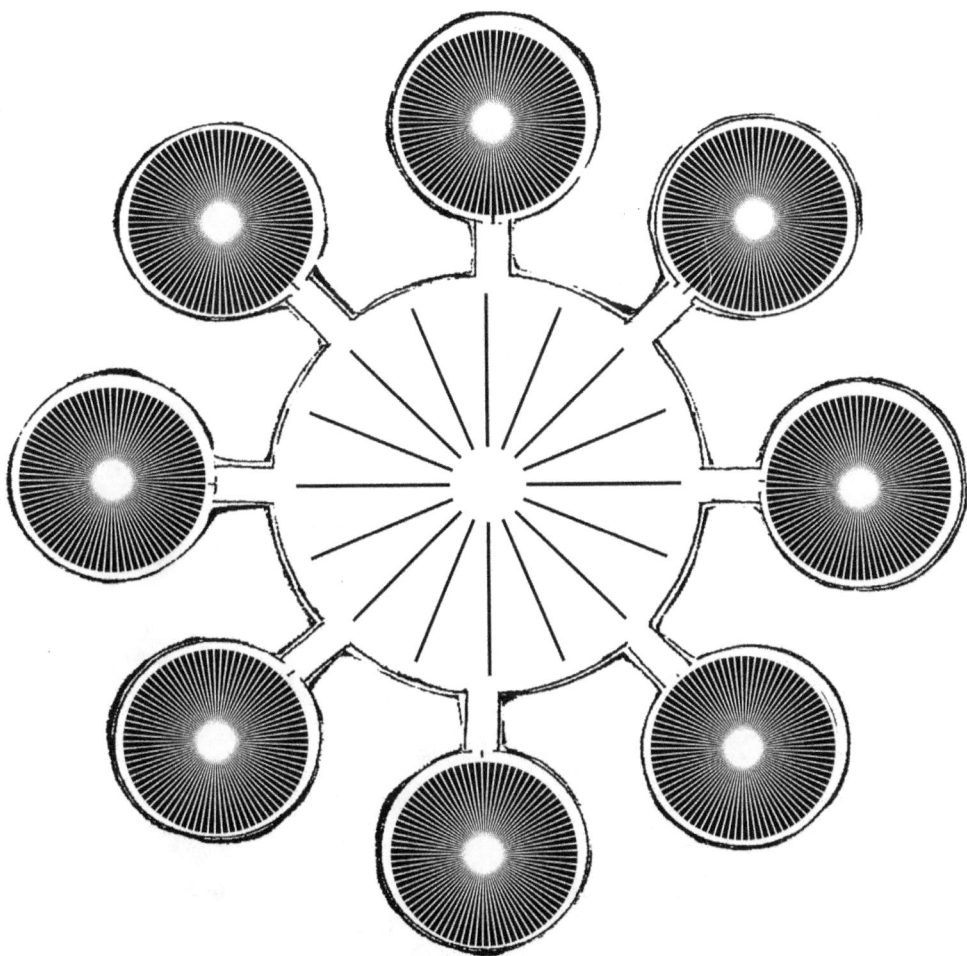

INTRODUCTION

THIS BOOK IS A SELF-HEALING PROJECT, dealing with simple things that we must do for our own well-being, along with learning to use the pendulum and divining rods to help get the answers you are looking for concerning your health, your environment and the way you live.

We are going to start from the position of the reader not knowing anything about dowsing. Let's be clear about one thing – anybody can dowse. All that has to happen is that you trust and let the dowsing tell you the result. When you dowse you are simply communicating with non-physical energy which is also part of us (we being the farthest extension of it). Since our thoughts create reality through the vibrational level they operate under, we must believe fully in what we are doing and keep our intention pure and focused – intention is our greatest source of power.

First impressions are lasting impressions: as a first step, once you have read this book, I hope you will be inspired to find a practising dowser to teach you or ask them if they know someone who can help. Dowsing picks up on your gut feeling and transmits the answer – in the form of a 'yes' or 'no' answer – to the pendulum. We are all able to access that part of ourselves which we call intuition, gut reaction, the higher truth, and once you learn to tap into that, all you have to do is practice, practice, practice.

The kind of healing that I am about to explain here is not a substitute for medical intervention but can hopefully work in conjunction. These pages contain a summary of my life experience along with my reading and personal research in over a decade of energetic healing work.

We are all born into this life to care for each other and for the earth. We have to start to understand that there is a big connection between disease, healing and personal power. Personal power is the foundation of health. Our power influences the body and spirit. By working with intuition and the diagnostic tools of higher wisdom, we can learn to identify the emotional and psychological causes of illness, for emotional and spiritual stresses are the root causes of all physical illness.

Cheer, hope, joy, love, and desire for health and happiness will mean healthy tissues, strong organs and good health in general. Fear, melancholy, malaise, hatred, dejection and loss of confidence will bring about a morbid state and the gradual depletion of organ function. We need to replace fear with confidence, courage and hope. "As a man thinketh in his heart, so is he" (*Book of Proverbs*, chapter 23, verse 7). Remember we cannot mis-experience anything in our lives – we can only misinterpret. In order to progress spiritually and allow healing in our lives we must trust the wisdom of our higher selves that we are at the right place and that goodness will prevail if we maintain an open, un-judgemental heart and attitude. Always believe in health and healing and speak to yourself – or the person being healed – as already well. Each time something bad happens, you have a choice how you react to it – you can take it as a learning experience or you can choose to be a victim. We are constantly creating our reality, and it is up to you if you create unconsciously/by default or with positive intention.

Whenever you call the vet, the first thing s/he asks is "What have you been feeding the animal on?". A doctor never asks that question and we have to ask ourselves why. We feed ourselves with the food that we eat, with the thoughts that we create and with the information we consume.

Illnesses fall into three types:
Acute, Temporary, Chronic

Acute disease can be life threatening and you may decide to see an allopathic doctor for emergency treatment and alleviation of symptoms rather than use complementary methods of treatment.

Temporary conditions will be alleviated by the whole immune system, given enough time. Such conditions need methods of treatment that work in harmony with that defence system and our body.

Chronic conditions throw up a more difficult problem. The body enters a locked state and is unable to break free of illness. Conventional medicine will often only alleviate symptoms, at best. There will most likely be a steady degeneration of health over time, so we need the key to unlock the system and allow recovery. It is the body's system that produces recovery, but the right therapies can lend a helping hand.

Universal Healing

We all know that Jesus was a great healer. This very fact was the founding idea behind Mary Baker Eddy's Church of Christ, Scientist. Jesus' method of healing was to deny the reality of the outward appearance, instead affirming only the inner perfection of the sufferer. This method is used today by successful practitioners, with the treatment taking place wholly in their minds. They do not heal by the use of willpower, nor do they influence the mind of the patient. The founding principle is that the practitioner believes the client to be perfect and then removes any idea that the client is unwell, using the Cosmic Intelligence. The patient comes in as a sick person but the practitioner must think of them as totally well in order to get through the mind barrier of illness. As soon as the patient substitutes his sick thoughts for the healer's perfect thought, the healing will begin.

This is the way Jesus healed, with no reliance on concentration, willpower, suggestion, hypnosis, etc. He used the power of the mind and set a positive mental intention in order to heal. Mind moulds the body. Understand the Law of Mind and you realise that the source of energy is infinite. Faith will then follow knowledge, because the more you know about healing the greater the faith you have in it. There are no sacred writings required in this process.

A mental and spiritual treatment is completed in the mind of the healer, who starts by thinking the patient is perfect in the Mind of God. At no time does the healer think of the patient as ill, but rather acts at all times to erase any belief in physical distortion by the client. The healer knows that we are all one mind and that both a sick mind and a well mind cannot be in the same place together. The intent is to merge the patient's mind with the healer's and with the Higher Power of the healer's mind in order to change the patient's way of thinking, and restore health.

The first step is total relaxation, both physical and mental, so that the healer and the patient join in one mind. The sick person thinks s/he has separated from God, but the fact remains that spirit can never be sick, therefore sickness has no law to support it. So, the healer must not devote too much time to the disease, for it has no basis. The more we look at it, or discuss it, the more false reality we put into it. We must only pay enough attention to it so as to be able to treat it. Remove all doubts about healing before healing starts, allowing the spirit to sweep through and cleanse every cell.

"The father in me, He it is that doeth the work. Of myself I can do nothing" (John 5:19). Whether you are a Christian or a member of any other faith, remember that we are not responsible for the healing and no credit is sought when healing is given. It is God (the Sacred Masculine and Feminine at the root of all religions) who provides the healing.

It is time that we understand the true destiny of humankind – not to live in sickness and suffering, not to be limited by physical illness. We are born for a higher destiny and we must live up to that, always seek the higher truth and don't be content with anything less.

David Willocks, Christchurch, NZ

www.selfhealingcentre.com

SIX PATHWAYS TO HEALTH

In his various books on health, the chemist Raymond Francis (*Never Be Sick Again; The Great American Health Hoax*) links all disease to malfunctioning cells, which occur either because of deficiency or toxicity. He identifies six pathways from disease to health:

1. Nutritional

Even in a world where people are richer and more comfortable than they have perhaps ever been in recent history, many people in our society suffer malnourishment. This is not because they don't eat enough but that they eat the wrong stuff; food deficient in nutrients. In our finely balanced bodies, the shortage of just one nutrient affects the entire system. Westerners in particular are very often overfed, yet undernourished. Fast food and processed food will leave us nutritionally deficient and chemically toxic. It is not an exaggeration to say that modern food promotes disease.

2. Through toxicology

Toxic exposure is a fact of life and the body is designed to deal with it, however, problems occur when there is a toxic overload. To find the culprits, we have to consider the air we breathe, the water we drink, the clothes we put onto our skin, and of course the food we eat. We know that in many places on earth both the air and the drinking water is polluted, and along with this there are the dangers of man-made fibres which contain toxic material (and hinder the body from sweating and regulating its heat in a natural way). We have already discussed the toxicity of food stuffs in the point before.

The body can detox, but it needs the essential nutrients to do this, and if you have poor digestion or don't get adequate exercise, then the body isn't functioning at its optimum level and therefore cannot detox properly. Add to this a mental diet of negative thoughts and emotions, and you can see how the stage is set for disease.

Excessive toxic exposure causes disease: reduce exposure by recognising the causes and avoid toxins on all levels.

3. Psychological

The mind has a huge effect on our health, and therefore it is imperative that we understand how thoughts, emotions and behaviour affect us.

Our mind is the driver of our entire body, with control over the brain and many of our functions. Although not openly and rationally discussed very often, the placebo effect, miraculous healings and spontaneous recoveries are part of everyday life and always have been. We already know that stress causes illness and that meditation helps our well-being. What we think or feel plays a major role in health and illness and may well be even more important than all the other pathways put together.

4. Physical

We need to understand how to provide for our bodies' physical needs on a daily basis, as a matter of routine. We can easily enhance our physical potential by doing the things that should come naturally to us: walking, eating healthily, getting adequate exercise and exposure to sunlight. On top of this, we should keep an eye on minimizing physical damage to our bodies through over-strain.

5. Genetic

Modern medicine has latched on to genetics as one of its champion causes for some diseases. However, it is not the primary cause of disease some would have you believe. Genes express themselves in a way commensurate with life's circumstances and a person can commit themselves to optimizing health, rather than accepting their genetic fate. Each human being is unique, not a generic genetic code: keep this in mind and optimize your genetic potential by promoting your own health. Your health belongs to you.

6. Medical

This is one of the most misunderstood of all pathways. A lot of people swear by modern medicine, and its advances in many areas should not be underplayed. However, it is becoming increasingly clear that the modern medical system offers very few cures; focusing instead on the suppression of symptoms, which can lead to unforeseen side-effects. While often excellent in a crisis and cases of trauma (painkillers, antibiotics, surgery for ruptured organs or broken bones), blind trust in allopathic doctors and their treatments (non-emergency surgery and drugs) to the exclusion of all other remedies and health systems can be destructive, or at the very least blocks a patient off from the very real benefits of systems that can work in harmony with the body in order to cure and promote long-term health.

In some cases, modern medicine can actually cause disease, and we must identify and avoid these potentially harmful aspects.

• • •

In conclusion, we need new theories for this new millennium. Modern diets, our nutritional intake, toxic exposure and stress levels bear little resemblance to the past of our species. Every cell in the body is affected, which is why we have so much chronic disease. The diseases we face today are a result of decades of inadequate nutrition, toxic exposure, sedentary lifestyle, family and social disruption and the mass dependency on drugs (both prescription and recreational).

Fountain of Youth

First and foremost, one must come to the understanding that the body cures itself. Allopathic and alternative medicine and healing techniques are there to help the patient heal themselves.

We have been searching for the fountain of youth for centuries, which basically means we have been constantly looking for a healthy way of living. Yet our present high-performance life, both productive and competitive, puts stresses on our bodies and minds and becomes the number one killer. While we spend millions on medical expenses, we seem to accept that there may not be any sure-fire way of getting better.

We must wake up and realise that we have the answer to our own health.

If the doctors said to you "Go home, exercise, eat healthily, cut down on alcohol, and get plenty of rest and sleep" you would think you were cheated, because they didn't give you a prescription, even though the advice they gave was the best one. All you had to do was follow it. Your body, mind, and soul are the greatest self-healing unit there is. All you have to do is keep your body ready to do the healing. Keep healthy and keep fit. Nature both creates and restores what has been created. The reason for disease is being out of harmony with God and nature.

The health of the body is in the blood, with the correct red and white cell balance and viscosity, and good circulation equals good health. If the blood is imbalanced or inhibited it will bring on disease, meaning a body out of balance. Knowing that the body restores and heals itself and that most people recover we then look to see why some people don't make it. If we look a bit deeper, we find that most of these people are tense and lead pressured lives and are unable to relax and release stress. Relaxation should become their first priority.

Royal Rife (famous for his work in radionics and dowsing) said "In reality, it is not the bacteria or virus that produce the disease but the chemical constituent of these micro-organisms enacting upon the unbalanced cell metabolism of the human body that in actuality produce the disease. We also believe if the metabolism of the human body is perfectly balanced or poised, it is susceptible to no disease."

Our body consists of billions of cells which are like minute batteries. Each cell has a positive end and a negative end (like a battery). Just like any battery-charged appliance, the cells must connect up positive to negative for the energies to flow. When the body's cells are balanced or polarised, tension is released and the mind and body are relaxed. When there is excess positive there is tension. When negative is in the excess and out of balance, fatigue follows. If there is an electrical leak, energy is depleted. These 'leaks' in our system can be caused by faulty thinking and living (at its most extreme – abuse or addiction).

Some degree of electrical imbalance is present in all mental and physical disorders, but when the entire body is out of balance, we have serious issues. In all cases the blood is affected and so is the blood flow through the body. Only when the balance is restored does the healing force start to work.

Leon Ernest Eeman was born in Belgium in 1889 and served in the First World War between 1915 and 1918, which left him with injuries from a plane crash, dysentery and malaria. During his lengthy recovery in hospital, Eeman conceived of a healing technique that utilized what he called "human radiations" or electric currents present in the body, what we now know as bioelectricity. His methods sought to balance or polarise the body, stopping electrical leaks and conserving energy, He knew that the body must act to known electrical laws, concluding that there must be positive/negative poles. When the electrical flow between positive and negative is not in balance we have disease. When the unbalanced condition is normalised, tension goes and body can commence healing.

There are positive and negative points on the human body. For a start, the head is positive, whereas the sacral is negative. Eeman would run a cable, with copper mats attached to either end, placing one under head and the other end under the sacrum (position of the sacral chakra – see chapter 'Faith is the Opposite of Fear'), thus connecting positive and negative between these two powerful points to connect the electrical field of the body. When opposite poles are connected together, they are known as the Eeman circuit.

There are different pole points all over the body, and once you become proficient in dowsing, you will be able to identify them yourself. Eeman's methods brought benefit to many sufferers of insomnia, neurasthenia, high blood pressure, abdominal problems, indigestion, and various mental conditions, as well as neuritis, rheumatism, moodiness, fever, asthma, respiratory and urinary tract problems and more.

MAINTAINING HEALTH ON A DAILY BASIS

*"You can't stop the waves,
but you can learn to swim."*

Jon Kabat-Zinn

To protect against disease, we need a strong immune system – we need to learn how to balance and to protect it so that it is always doing its job optimally. A strong system does not mean an overactive one, it is a balanced system that we need, neither overactive nor underactive. Many people who have infections, or even those with cancer, can attribute their illness to a weakening of the immune system that is brought on by negativity, stress or even inappropriate medical treatment.

Allopathic medicine sees infection and cancer in terms of a war; as intruders which must be beaten back with weapons, even if they happen to be poisons. While killing the 'invaders' these treatments often harm the immune system at the same time, weakening our innate ability to fight and heal ourselves. If instead of trying to destroy the infection or cancer, we built up our immune system, we would be more effective at controlling disease. After all, it's your immune system that determines your health and even how you will die. If kept in optimum condition, it will protect you against viruses, bacteria, yeast, fungi, parasites and toxins.

Successful health care relies on preventing disease and raising the body's healing power. A balanced immune system means we get enough of some things and not too much of others, since weaknesses in our immune systems can be brought about by nutritional deficiency/excesses, poor digestion or eating too much of the same type of foods, as well as virus or bacterial overload, toxins and chemicals.

The immune system is your own personal army, naturally protecting you twenty-four hours a day, seven days a week, destroying and removing viruses, bacteria, yeast, tumours and toxins. The two major cells operating in the immune system are macrophages and lymphocytes, both white blood cells. These are the white blood cells that search and destroy unhealthy cells in the body.

Surveillance, defence and housekeeping are the duties of the immune system. Surveillance is constant, happening all the time even in healthy people: the location and destruction of tumours and other issues happen as soon as they arise in healthy people. If our immune system is strong, we can resist the onset of disease.

The defence function of a healthy immune system is always fighting against infectious organisms. We are constantly being attacked by infections which will not develop into a disease because our immune system is able to deal with it in good time.

As for the housekeeping function of a healthy immune system, this too is of utmost importance. It is there to clean up the old cells in the body and remove them, rather like a vacuum cleaner.

To help your immune system stay strong you need to eat nutrient-dense foods, including green leafy vegetables, yellow vegetables, cereals, seeds, nuts, fruits and berries. You need a good balance of vitamins and minerals. You also need good digestion to process all this healthy food, as this reduces any allergic reactions you might have. A sensible plan would be to mix different types of food in your diet and avoid eating just the same foods every day.

There has never been a time in history that the immune system has needed more attention. We need to find a methodology of maintaining a healthy system based on simple safe alternatives and natural means to treat minor problems. Interesting and valuable insights have been gained in preventing cancer through balancing your immune system. We must keep our immune system in top class order through the regular practise of good diet, exercise and a healthy mental attitude.

Viruses, Bacteria, Cancer

You may well be surprised to know that none of these are the bad guys, despite the fear associated with their names. They are – and always have been – a part of our lives. They are the cleaners and the sanitation workers who – like in our cities – are part of the daily work of keeping the environment of our bodies clear of rubbish and the bad stuff that can create disease. Viruses, bacteria and cancer cells sit inside us all the time, waiting to eat up the weak and dying cells in our bodies when necessary, recycling only the sick and dying.

If our body is healthy and clean there is nothing to recycle so viruses, bacteria and cancer cells actually don't do anything – they are simply present and waiting for when the body needs them. And this is where diet comes in – if we eat the wrong foods, foods that disrupt the balance of Ph acidity in the body, that is where things start to go wrong. Sugary, processed or dead food like meat will make the body's Ph acidic, and the first signs of an imbalance may well be any itching on the skin, or a yeast infection (candida). The next sign would be smelly gas and runny stools, which, when you think about it, are an indication that something is rotting inside of you. These symptoms are like the internal rust in a car, which will eventually spread to the mainframe.

So don't blame cancer cells, they're only doing their job!

Viruses, bacteria and cancer cells only turn against us when there is a weakness in our body, mind or soul. Just as you have to take great care over what you ingest into your wonderful body, you also have to be careful about what you what you say, how you think, and what emotions you keep in your heart. Negativity can eat you up, your survival depends on looking on the Bright Side, walking on the Bright Side and keeping yourself close to the Bright Side.

Anger, anxiety, resentment, fear, jealousy, hatred and even excessive sadness can all create negative affirmations in our words and actions. Stop feeling sorry for yourself. It will kill you. Don't put other people down, for the negative effect will come back on you.

Everybody lives in fear of something, be it fear of poverty, ill health, death, fear of lost love, of old age, or fear of criticism. Most fears are inherited and they must be mastered to advance in this life. As you practise and gain expertise, you can find out or dowse for how many fears you have and which ones you need to conquer. All of our fears can be healed by balancing energy levels and altering thoughts from past events.

The Power of Thought

It can well be hard to believe that the power of thought can affect living organisms such as bacteria and viruses. Psychic healers believe the presence of bacteria and viruses in the body's system is perfectly natural and healthy. It is only when there is an imbalance between good and bad bacteria and viruses that disease occurs.

Orthodox medicine considers the cause of most disease to be because of invasion from outside of us, although this assumption has never been proven. Psychic healing works from the inside, helping the body's own defences overcome imbalances or invasions by activating them to their fullest capacity.

The thought commands create electrical forces that go into action wherever they are needed in the body.

Healthy cells maintain a balance between positive and negatively charged particles within the cell itself; it is through this balance that we achieve polarity. The polarity of positive and negative allow the energy to flow through the body constantly. When polarity is upset, the entire system suffers, because this is the life force and operating power which allows humans to function on a physical, mental and spiritual level.

Proper, healthy living habits simply come down to a way of life in which positive and negative forces are maintained. At the very minimum, this demands a person have the correct amount of rest and sleep, along with adequate physical exercise. A balanced diet, minimal artificial stimuli from drugs alcohol and tobacco. This does not mean that a glass of wine will kill you, but alcohol per se is not conducive to the harmonious way of life. It comes down to this: all disease is caused by improper thinking. The presence of toxic substances in the system is due to the fact that one is ignorant of these dangers and thus guilty of making uninformed decisions.

Much is said about the healing power of love. Seen through the eyes of a psychic healer, love is a strong positive electric force, created in the emotional system of one person and directed towards one or more other individuals. This positive energy may be a message that is a personal desire to share, unite physically and mentally, or it may be the desire to bring various values to a large segment of the population. Love is probably the maximum potential power that an individual is capable of generating within themselves.

Conversely, hatred can create a parallel negative force. Even frustration or the inability to express oneself can lead to physical manifestations through various diseases. However, disease is not necessarily connected with area of frustration, as a frustrated lover does not develop heart disease or malfunctions of the sexual organs.

The issue with frustration is that, if it has no outlet outside the system, it turns within itself and causes havoc wherever the system is weakest.

Everyone's system has a certain weak point where an attack will yield the most severe results. Since there is no way of telling which way it will go, diagnosis is difficult. But, if we eliminate the particular frustration that causes illness by simply changing the circumstances, we would enable instant healing! Since most frustrations do not yield that easily, we might work on trying to change a person's attitude towards his frustration, thereby allowing energies liberated from the frustration to flow into more constructive channels. Fear causes both mental and physical illness.

When tackling fear, we must remember that it is connected to the person's absence of information as to why they feel that way. If we can pinpoint the fear, we then need to get as much information to the person about its cause in order to deal with it. The fear will dissolve once the truth of the circumstances which have initiated it have been identified, explained and integrated by the person on the mental, emotional/body and spiritual level.

Diet

You are what you eat has a great deal of truth to it. It is not the amount of food or combination of food we eat, but the quality of ingested nutrients that is significant. Diet in relation to healing should be more of a preventive attitude towards nutrition, combined with avoidance of that food that encourages disease. Try to avoid, or at least reduce, foods that are damaging to health, such as cola drinks, the majority of sodas, white sugar, ice-cream, white bread and processed food in general.

One might also say, however, that it is not just what you eat but how you chew and digest the food, as well as your mood when eating.

Food may be harmless when eaten in a relaxed state but if it is eaten while we are upset or anxious, then it can have the wrong effect on the body. Never eat after an argument or when dealing with bad news, as the digestion will not work as it should. It is always best to calm down and relax so that you can then appreciate your food in an appropriately positive state of mind. Totally withdraw from your problems for a moment before eating.

Toxins

Do you know why you feel sluggish and tired? These are signs that there are toxins in your body, which appear in the form of parasites that find ways in to your brain and organs.

To give your system a clear-out, take 2 tsp Epsom Salts in some water and make sure that for the rest of the day you remain close to a toilet. No matter the state of your health, follow this healing and you will be alright.

Fasting

Fasting is an easy way to clean your system. Simply stop eating at 8 pm in the evening and don't start eating again till as close to midday the following day as you can manage. While you are fasting, drink water and juices to keep yourself hydrated. You will feel hungry and you may well start to feel sick or even experience some pain. However, stay focused on the task and resist eating for the entire period.

Exercise

Exercise involves at least thirty minutes of reasonably strenuous activity for five days a week. It's best to feel a little puffed after such exercise, not to overdo it with tough regimes that will leave you exhausted, but to increase gradually.

Rest & Relaxation

We all suffer from stress in some form. High blood pressure, stomach ulcers, or sheer exhaustion. People who are too stressed are harming their immune system and leaving themselves prone to infection. We need at least one day of total rest a week. Plus, a two-week holiday every year. Aim for eight hours in bed every night, as the benefits of this are great.

Alternative Therapies

Dr Lawrence Sanson has outlined a selection for maintaining everyday health in an effective way. We will outline these here, without going into great detail, which you can explore independently.

Selenium: low levels of selenium can render a person prone to disease.
Garlic: The ancient Egyptians used garlic widely and so have many civilisations since. It stimulates our immune system especially against colds and flu and intestinal infections.
Echinacea: this boosts the immune system and prevents viral infection.
Buccaline Berna: this is taken at the beginning of winter and three months later. It is an oral vaccine to prevent bacterial complications

Enzogenol: this comes from pine bark and is a powerful antioxidant. It insures an enhanced state of well-being as well as a greater resistance to infections.

Tea Tree Oil: this is derived from Melaleuca alternifolia which is antibacterial. Taken orally it can heal stomach ulcers.

Ginko: for 5000 years the Chinese have used the leaves of this tree to aid memory. Western medicine has taken an interest in Ginko because it aids longevity. It can also be very beneficial to people with cold hands and feet. If you regularly take Aspirin or Warfarin, you should not use Ginko.

Ginseng: used for thousands of years by the Chinese to boost immunity.

St John's Wort: helps greatly with anxiety and is a natural antidepressant. Good to use as a pick-me-up after illness.

Valerian: night time sedative and free of side effects.

Aspirin: good for relief of pain and fever.

Iron: used for producing Haemoglobin in the blood which transports oxygen around the body. A balanced diet should provide adequate iron.

Calcium: needs to be in the diet and levels in the body need to be checked by a doctor in later life.

Flavonoids: these form a large group of naturally occurring antioxidants that stimulate the immune system and help with prevention of degenerative processes.

Homocysteine: this is an amino acid produced by the body which needs to be kept in balance as high levels can cause dementia, osteoporosis, failing eyesight. Again, they can best be controlled by diet. Both vitamins B6 and B12 act as cofactors for enzymes that break down potent homocysteine to innocuous amino acid (see below).

Essential vitamins: Vitamin B complex; Vitamins A, D, and E; Vitamin C.

Colloidal Silver

Colloidal Silver is one of the most powerful natural antibiotics there is. It has been used for thousands of years for health and prevention of disease in humans and also in the preservation and storage of food. In the times of European settlement of America, the settlers would put a silver coin in a bucket of milk to make it keep, and it is said that the aristocracy of Europe used silverware in order to protect themselves from the effects of bad food or bacteria.

Today colloidal silver is the most convenient way to use the beneficial qualities of silver, and it is way cheaper and easier to make than ever before. Because of the low cost and ease of production, more people should be using colloidal silver today.

Colloidal silver is an antibiotic that kills all types of virus, fungus, and bacteria. It is also perfectly harmless: non-toxic to all livings things that are not single-celled. Single-celled life forms such as viruses, fungus and bacteria rely on oxygen-metabolising enzymes to survive. Colloidal silver cuts off the oxygen-metabolism, causing the pathogen to die within six minutes. Basically, colloidal silver cripples the chemical lung of single-celled pathogens through suffocation.

While there may be side effects with man-made antibiotics, colloidal silver only reacts with the oxygen of the pathogen. Since pathogens have not been able to build up resistance to colloidal silver because of its fast reaction, six minutes from contact, there is no chance of the resistance – and therefore inefficacy – that affect so many common antibiotics in use today.

Colloidal silver is manufactured at 5 ppm (parts per million) or more, using two 99 % silver wires and a 27 volt adapter which you can plug into the mains, and preferably distilled water. You will also need a plastic holder for the 2 silver wires, which must be kept parallel in the water, and a glass jar of distilled water. These units are easily available and mean you can make the colloidal silver yourself. Once you have paid the initial set-up cost, the cost of making it is very small. The only other thing you may want to invest in is a meter that tells you the levels of impurity (ppm) in the water. The meter is used to measure the ppm in the water before you start, and to check it later to see that you have added 5 ppm of silver on top of the previous ppm you started with.

Dr William Stewart Halsted wrote of colloidal silver, in 1913: "I know of nothing that could take its place ... We have only scratched the surface of silver's medical brilliance. Already it's an amazing tool. It stimulates bone-forming cells, cures the most stubborn infections of all kinds, and stimulates in skin and other soft tissues."

Varied uses include, acne, cuts, eczema, rash, warts, digestion, parasites. diarrhoea, healing crisis. It can also be used for water purification and added to food products such as mayonnaise, dairy products and left overs, in order to extend the life of the product. Use with pets and also in their housing and surroundings, since they often suffer from parasites, which attack and eat the body cells of the host, excreting their waste into the hosts' tissues and bloodstream. Colloidal silver selects only those disease-causing pathogens and suffocates them.

The recommended daily dose is 1tsp per adult to begin with, and 1/2 tsp for children, increasing after approximately 4 weeks. If a person is suffering from any illness, the dose should be increased to 1 tsp 3 times a day per adult, and 1/2 tsp 3 times a day for children. In the eventuality of an outbreak of major disease, you would increase the dose significantly, up to three times this amount. Allow four days of treatment in order to feel the benefit of the colloidal silver. It accumulates in the body and like any healthy cell it is continually being replaced. If illness is chronic, it is best to take the higher dose. Taking sufficient colloidal silver daily prevents infection, disease, and even reduces toxicity in skin burns (helps with healing). It can be viewed as your second immune system, giving valuable help in the immune system's workload, eradicating pathogens in the body. Colloidal silver acts in parallel with the immune system but not in conjunction. As a preventive, colloidal silver is easy to use and an effective disease fighter.

Storage: keep colloidal silver in a food storage area, away from electrical appliances. Store in a coloured glass jar or bottle away from the sun. Because colloidal silver is electrically charged it does not keep well in plastic. Do not store in refrigerator or freezer.

Ideal to have in a pandemic, for contaminated water or air, germ warfare and military activity (in case of anthrax or lesser causes, colloidal silver could be a life-saver). Low levels of silver in the body can lead to being prone to colds, flu, fevers, and other chronic illnesses. Colloidal silver works on a wide range of pathogens and has no side effects nor does it cause damage to healthy cells in the host's body.

Ulric's Way: New Zealand's Greatest Doctor

Ulric Williams is regarded as New Zealand's greatest doctor. During the late 1930s, he was having issues with the medical profession ridiculing him, even as he watched his patients suffer more than they should have. Not only was the medical system plundering the people, he noticed, but the banks and churches were doing it too. He saw eighty percent of the medical system as nothing but cruel, ludicrous, and a transparent fraud, considering that doctors knew nothing about disease, nothing about natural cures, and nothing about spiritual provisions for maintaining or regaining good health.

Sound familiar? The situation we find ourselves in today is not new – all this has already been done to us, and has been playing out for the past eighty or ninety years. It seems that there will continue to be suffering until people start to take responsibility for their own health. Someday soon we are all going to need each other. Don't worry about the future, it's not going to be more of the same, if we stick together, it will be better. It is futile to blame the collapse of our society on our medical personnel, bankers or clergy. Only Divine intervention will allow disease, disaster, brutality and violence to give way to health, prosperity, security and deliverance from darkness and despair.

The word doctor comes from the Latin, 'to teach'. It is a doctor's job to teach other people to be well, the doctor is not the person that heals you. All the doctor does is teach you to heal yourself and using this principle and spirit of God, you are able to treat yourself – hopefully for the rest of your life.

Williams advocated these simple rules: not to eat when you are not hungry or when you are ill. Fast bi-monthly – from the last meal at night to at least past noon on the next day – and maybe supplement this by taking vitamin C with water. In this way, you remove toxins and waste from your body. Eat fresh food, exercise to increase oxygen, and as ever "Always think of yourself as being well."

Here are some of his quotes and advice Ulrich Williams gave to his patients, and which can still serve us today:

- You are what you think. You become what you think. To be healthy you must think in the right way. You have to think healthily and avoid filling your mind with predictions of bad things that may happen.
- Thoughts have a way of attracting to you what you think about.
- As a man thinketh in his heart, so he is.
- You are what you eat. If you put kerosene in your car you wouldn't expect it to run properly, so you can't expect your body to run well if you put rubbish in it.
- Commit yourself to clearing your system of toxins by eating well and maintaining an easy protocol of exercise, fresh air, good nutrition, regular elimination and healthy thoughts. Good health is up to you.
- God is love (the highest energy) – trust in him and only good things will happen.
- "Don't get your kids injected for whooping cough. It will only cause complaints later in life."
  (This is in the 1930s. Ask yourself if anything has changed.)

- One of his trusted cures for arthritis was to put one cup of baking soda and one cup of Epsom Salts in an evening bath. Go to bed afterwards as it will probably make you perspire (perhaps that is the cure). Repeat as necessary.
- Sore back – "You know you have got it in your mind that you're going to be in a wheelchair and it is colouring your mind. Stop thinking about the wheelchair and your back can right itself."
- He often used shock treatment. He once used very bad language against a client who had had a number of surgeries. When quizzed on this, he responded: "Oh well, the silly fool. He has already let them have his appendix. Now he is letting them have his gall-bladder, he won't listen to common sense."
- Lots of people use the medical service as a means to save themselves from pain and distress. If the doctor says "Let's see how we can change this lifestyle," he believed that half of them wouldn't come back.
- If you want to become good, be good. If you want to become well, eat well.
- All you have to do is to stand in your own light, and let the blessings come into you.
- Healing comes to those who want health and want to use it for right, not just for their own selfish ends.
- Don't say "Please, God" say "Thank you, Father."
- If you are well and want to stay well, half your food should be eaten raw. If you are sick and want to get better, three quarters of your food should be eaten raw.
- Faith means to expect a good outcome. Expect to be healed. Know that God can heal you. Faith is like posting a letter, you expect it to be delivered so you can then forget about it.
- When you pray, don't say "Please" say "Thank you".
- The body can mimic any disease that has ever made a strong and frightening impression on the person's mind.

- If someone comes to you and says "I am trying to get better," you must say "I don't want you to try, I want you to do it. You are going downhill! I want you to turn around and go uphill and not to say 'I'll try!'"
- No disease is incurable, but some patients are, because they don't want to change. They go to their death like sheep to slaughter, just because they will not change.
- You don't have to do anything to get better, all you need is to stop doing what is wrong. If you want to know what that is, your divine intelligence will tell you. Your body has a healing power that will heal you when you stop making yourself sick.
- Use the power of the body to heal itself and remove conditions that make you sick.
- Put some spirituality in your life with Love, Faith and Forgiveness.
- The secret to health is what you put in your mouth, the exercise you give your body and the thoughts you have in your mind.
- Envy means you have a mental picture of lacking the things you desire. This belief in lack perpetuates lack. Picture yourself having the thing you desire and it will happen.
- Anything you think or say with belief and conviction will come true. Change your thinking, change your life. All chronic disease is a mental habit.
- "All is well" "All is well" "All is well". Whenever you feel pain in your body say to yourself repeatedly "All is well".

Williams asserted that disease is a slow degenerating process, caused firstly by failure to fulfil the requirements of well-being and then by attempts at prevention and cure. Disease begins with an inner toxic and/or deficient condition ('failure to fulfil the requirements of well-being') which is then exacerbated by external toxins and through the attempts to cure in ways which further depletes vitamins and minerals. For him, healing was a gradual regenerative process relying on the self-cleaning mechanisms of the body, but before you can be healed you must be cleansed. Management not treatment of acute illness is what is called for. We are the only animals that haven't got the sense to stop eating when we are sick.

In a well-known case, he treated a lady with cancer of the bladder, who had been told that no further treatment was possible. She was put on a strict diet and warned that there would be a healing crisis. A sudden worsening of symptoms and fever, vomiting and diarrhoea followed, and she was instructed that when this happened, she was to stop eating food, go on a citrus juice and water diet, rest and have an enema every day. This simple and effective treatment brought on a complete cure.

These are treatments and methods crying out for recognition that are so simple and effective. Most medics are worried about people doing their own healing and will do everything to promote what they have been taught at medical school. What we need is a selfcare healthy nation of people not a forever-sickness system sustaining the pharmaceutical industry.

The power that heals us is within us. Rarely does the healing power within us need any help. All it needs is a fair chance and the necessary conditions. So many people around the world have been given the prognosis: "there is nothing more we can do for you", or are going through treatment that is expensive, useless or worse. The majority of these could get better if they lived obediently and handed over control to the power within. Trust in the ability of the power within and sensible living to stop causing disease – this is the key to success.

The life force within is the only thing that can make and keep us well. It will almost always succeed if we give it a chance. We just have to remove the barriers, psychological and physical, even if that means admitting that you have to end a relationship in order to be true to yourself, for there is no personal goal higher than the maintenance of your own health and balance. Clear your mind of emotional barriers like fear, resentment, worry, self-pity, jealousy, pride, greed, gluttony, lust, together with negative thoughts, beliefs, suggestions and impressions that the mind is acting on. These are by far the worst causes of disease. Disease in most cases is the effect of the mind's imprint on the body. Quit trying to get rid of your symptoms, since they will simply be taken away when the cause has been removed. The life force heals from within, sustains, protects and plans. Give it complete control.

Another vital aspect here is faith: faith is not some abstruse theological formula that neither the purveyor nor victim can understand. Faith is expectation. To regain lost health, we must stop making ourselves sick through lack of faith. Have faith and refrain from behaviour and thoughts that make you sick.

Why all this disease, you may ask, well, some people actually want to remain sick, to draw attention to themselves, feel important, to dominate, or out of laziness or revenge, or because the economy is organised to make and keep them ignorant, sick, terrified and exploitable. To become good, we must be good. To become well, we must start now. Healthy people do not suffer from and cannot be infected with TB or cancer. The real cause is dead food, stale air, and negative emotional states. Wake up, this is what is happening today!

Williams warned us in the 1930s about the "Bug Wallahs" in New Zealand's Department of Disease who were out to compel everyone to submit to periodic x-rays for TB. He saw it as a power trip, with those individuals wanting to rule over the x-ray machines, order treatments, and consign you to an exercise camp at their pleasure.

This reminds us that in the 1970s Sweden undertook a ten-year campaign to offer free testing for cervical cancer. However, they soon stopped it because the death rate didn't go down, but instead increased. Fear is a huge factor in creating disease. Stress damages the immune system and probably the worst stress is fear. Screening actually turns out to be dangerous, because it focuses the mind on disease when it should be focusing on health.

Wouldn't it be wonderful if instead of disease-oriented hospitals there were Health Homes to help people to help each other, and themselves.

BALANCE AND HIGH VIBRATION

"Science is tending to show that life is harmony – a state of being in tune – and that disease is discord or a condition when a part of the whole is not vibrating in union."

EDWARD BACH

High Vibrations and the pH Balance

We don't talk much about vibration, but every living thing that exists is vibrating. Even the trees, standing tall on their trunks, are actually moving in their extremities all the time. So it is with us – our thoughts are the wind through our leaves and branches. Negative thoughts operate on a low vibration and can therefore give you disease. Positive thoughts operate at a high vibration and can rid you of disease. It is our positive thoughts that maintain our wellness.

We have to remember that words have power – they are the manifestation of our thoughts into the physical world around us. And therefore, it makes sense that we have to be careful about what we say or what we listen to. Words have power, and in this world of ours there are many people who talk in a negative way, increasing our fear and subsequently increasing body stress.

When the body is in stress, it creates an acidic environment which activates the viruses, bacteria and cancer cells inside us to work overtime, and illness follows.

Stress affects every cell in the body and turns them from their natural alkaline state to an acidic state. Our body functions on the Acid – Alkaline pH Scale. Blood needs to be more alkaline than acid: on a scale of 0 acid ---- 14 alkaline, the ideal average would be 7.4. Improper pH balance leads to illness and disease; the blood must not be too acidic or alkaline, either extreme is dangerous.

So how to turn body pH from acid to alkaline?

Shut off the TV and most of the news outlets; they are toxic because they are built on the intention to ignite sensation, create fear and encourage addiction (more fear creates the need for more news, which causes rising acidity in us that we mistakenly feed with more fear). The endless bad news we hear from the media, the worst-case scenarios and predictions, all feed us fear and add to our feelings of powerlessness and insecurity. Focus on what you know.

The body's acid-alkaline balance is a key component of health. The Royal Free Hospital and School of Medicine in London concluded that raising one's pH (to an alkaline state) increases the immune system's ability to kill bacteria. Viruses and bacteria, which cause illnesses such as bronchitis and the common cold, thrive on acid. Our pH levels need to be slightly alkaline in the 6.7 to 7.2 range.

Dr Otto Warburg, doctor and Nobel Prize winner, states that "No disease can exist in an alkaline environment." Dr Warburg's recipe to help make the body more alkaline, reinvigorate the system, curb sore throats and restore the balance of stomach acid, bad digestion, tooth ache, kidney and urinary issues:

» 2 tablespoons freshly squeezed lemon or apple cider vinegar.

» 1/3 teaspoon of baking soda.

» Mix ingredients well, it will then start to fizz.

» Continue to add in more baking soda till it stops fizzing.

» Pour in 250 ml water and drink at once.

You can measure your pH levels with pH strips which are dipped in either saliva or urine and then checked against a colour chart. Testing urine first thing in the morning gives a good indication of whether your supplement or diet programme is alkaline enough. If you find that your pH is regularly below 6.4, it means that the body is too acidic and is low on mineral reserves. If this state continues, the immune system suffers.

Stress

Stress lies behind every illness known to us. It eats you up. Those feelings that you are hiding or holding back are acidic and will literally eat holes in you. Some feelings and memories are trapped behind our trauma self defence system, meaning we cannot access them because they have been hidden from us by internal mechanisms of the psyche in order to save us from pain. Therefore, we have to find a way to access them in order to liberate ourselves from their power through various health and healing techniques: there are plenty on offer in the field of yoga, meditation, hypnotherapy and Emotional Freedom Technique (EFT), etc.

The only way to liberate yourself from those negative, stressful feelings is to face them, deal with them and then to let them go. To free yourself of corrosive issues and free them from your system. The negative energy of negative thoughts must go somewhere, and you don't want them to go into your own body, thereby poisoning it. This is the reason why you have to identify them, deal with them and then eject them from your system. For whatever we think, we attract.

Laugh for no reason and smile, the sun will shine tomorrow and the world is old and has lived through many stages and events. We can trust it to continue in its magnificent beauty.

Make others happy and help those you can, for these positive deeds – done in the right spirit of love and selflessness – will bring positivity into your life. Just be careful that you love yourself too and that you are not sacrificing yourself to fulfil some guilt complex or sense of unworthiness. The most important thing is to be honest with yourself and understand your motivation. Helping others and bringing happiness into their lives should come from that loving place inside you and be given for free. The return will come in the positivity you invite into your system through these positive acts and the energy they bring.

Negative thoughts and feelings, the ingestion of bad things, will cause illness. Get them out of your way and healing will happen.

Emotion, Mind and Soul

Feelings are much more powerful than we imagine. Your body is a reflection of how you feel inside. How you are thinking affects the body and then the body affects our feelings. As in every major religious teaching, our aim should be to be at peace with ourselves.

This doesn't mean we should hide our feelings though, as this will simply force the body to move the stress somewhere else, and we will suffer ulcers, headaches, cancers and tumours as the result of feelings and emotions not admitted to or worked out.

The cells in our body are like soldiers, ready to go to war for us! Remember that your body is yours and it works for you. It's on your side, so you have to take care of it, keep it fed with the right food and nourished with the right thoughts.

If you say 'I feel like shit and wish I could die', that is what your body hears. It will work for the intentions you have expressed, and if you express negative wishes like that, you may well end up with bowel problems and body cells that start ageing and dying.

If you let yourself suffer too long with a broken heart, without acknowledging it and allowing yourself time to grieve and to heal, then your heart will start to weaken. Thoughts are the most powerful healer or killer. And you are in the driving seat, deciding which road to take.

The Power
of Frequencies
to Heal Disease

Frequency is defined as a measurable rate of electrical energy that is constant between two points, which changes with our mood, our food and our environment (both inside and out). We are constantly influenced by the magnetic action of the frequencies that surround us each day, and these frequencies affect our health and well-being. Everything on this earth has an electrical frequency measured in Hertz – humans, animals, plants and even stones!

A healthy human body vibrates in the higher ranges. However, in our modern societies there are a lot of people who operate on low vibrational levels due to fatigue, emotional exhaustion, hypothermia, chronic disease, fear, blocked emotions and nervous tension.

The average frequency of the Earth today is about 27.4 Hz, but there are places which can be considered hubs of low frequency, such as hospitals, prisons, areas near power lines, airports, underground train systems, public electric vehicles, shopping centres and offices. In such places, the vibrational level is less than 20 Hz, well below that of the earth.

Just as with places, people can also lower their frequency through states of mind: those with inflated egos, whose wish is to control or those who live in fear, have low vibrations. To give you some example of low vibration rates: grief and fear come in at 0.1 to 2 Hz; resentment 0.6 to 3.3 Hz; anger: 1.4 Hz and pride: 0.8 Hz; neglect 1.5 Hz; sense of superiority: 1.9 Hz. It's clear to see that these levels are well below the earth average, and when compared to the frequencies of higher thought and emotion, can be shown to be so degrading to our systems: acts of generosity have frequencies of 95 Hz: Thanks is 45 Hz; gratitude 140 Hz; a feeling of unity, 144 Hz; compassion is 150+ (whereas as pity would be a mere 3 Hz); love is 50 Hz; being loved 150 Hz, and unconditional love is 205 Hz.

It becomes clear that a person who does not increase their vibrations is exposing themselves to illness and may soon leave the earth plane in one way or another. The choice is ours, and it is up to us to increase our own vibration. We must choose to vibrate on a higher frequency; vibrating feelings of love and a sense of joy, and in this way heal our wounds. It is our task to rid ourself of fear and anger and to release the emotions which lower our vibrations.

Gratitude comes from within, and it all comes down to an appreciation of abundance, positive thinking and feeling the love. We need to make sure we

To aid the process of increasing our personal vibrations, we can change our diet to concentrate on high-vibrational foods which are organic and unprocessed. We can also start using essential oils to aid our upliftment:
Rose is 320 MHz
Frankincense: 147 MHz
Lavender: 118 MHz
Chamomile: 105 MHz
Juniper: 98 MHz
Peppermint: 89 MHz

spend time with high vibration people, since we know that many people's frequency is the average of the people they associate with. Drinking plenty of good quality water, meditating or finding time for quiet relaxation in nature as well as exercising will help us. So will breathing deeply and getting the blood pumping.

The power of frequencies to heal disease:

These are energies that the body needs to operate at, for optimum health.

62–78 MHz	Body (whole)	67–70 MHz	Heart
72–90 MHz	Brain	58–65 MHz	Lungs
72–78 MHz	Neck up	55–60 MHz	Liver
60–68 MHz	Neck down	60–80 MHz	Pancreas
65–68 MHz	Thymus Gland		

Ailments:

57–60 MHz	Colds/Flu	52 MHz	Epstein Barr
58 MHz	Disease starts	42 MHz	Cancer
55 MHz	Candida	25 MHz	DEATH

Frequencies of food

Processed/Canned Food:	Zero
Fresh Produce:	15 MHz
Dried Food:	15–22 MHz
Fresh Herbs:	20–27 MHz

Keep the frequency of your body above 62 MHz by making sure your diet consists mainly of high-frequency foods, combining this with positive thought, fresh air and meditation. Food, thought, fitness and spiritual practice combined, will bring your body up to the optimal frequency for health.

If you avoid eating junk food, canned and processed foods, disease and micro-organisms will have a hard time surviving. Meditate on a daily basis as it increases the frequencies of your energies, even just for a brief period.

A Short Note on the Corona Virus

As we have stated before, everything on earth is vibrating, each at different frequencies. It stands to reason that certain frequencies can protect from disease, while other frequencies can invite disease into our bodies. Herein lies the link between frequency (vibration) and health. Scientific research has shown that different parts of our bodies have their own sonic signature, with the cells of your heart having different 'harmonics' than the sound of the cells of your lungs.

Each disease carries its own vibrational signature, and Corona is a low vibration virus with an enclosed structure of the electro-magnetic circuit. Its vibrational frequency ranges from approximately 5.5 Hz to 14.5 Hz, while in higher ranges it is not active. When the vibrational frequency goes over 25.5 Hz, the virus simply cannot survive. This means that people who maintain high vibrations are unlikely to catch the virus.

Lessons Through Illness

One thing must be understood: we are all the masters of our fate when it comes to illness. We are not victims or unfortunate recipients of the illnesses we manifest, but authors of the story. Our own consciousness in the world is led by the ego, which seeks control and power and is continually caught up in the story of our progress in the world, without the illusion of which it would feel powerless and senseless.

The state of our bodies is a barometer of the state of our consciousness. Everything that happens in the body is an expression of the corresponding programmes of information that we have learnt. Harmony = Health; Disturbance of Health = Illness. Ease and dis-ease. If a person's consciousness becomes imbalanced, then this will create tangible symptoms in the body. It is the mind and soul that chart the course to illness, not the body, which only responds.

Symptoms show up first within a person's consciousness. There are a vast number of symptoms that the body can manifest yet they are all expressions of the same event (illness) and always occur within the person's consciousness. When a symptom manifests in the body it draws attention to itself, demanding to be looked at and dealt with. We regard it mostly as a nuisance and something to be got rid of as soon as possible. And because we hate to be disturbed in our routine, we commence a battle against the symptom.

The basis of allopathic medicine goes along with the resistant thought patterns of the average patient, reinforcing the idea that a symptom is a more or less accidental phenomenon whose cause is to be sought in the medicinal processes available. With this mindset, they are condemning both symptom and illness to meaninglessness, taking away the function of meaning that each symptom is signalling. As so many allopathic medicines suppress symptoms, the meaning is also suppressed in us.

Vehicles have instrument panels and warning lights when a part of the car or truck or plane malfunctions. If the light comes on, you have to take notice and interrupt your journey for the sake of safety. These warning lights are the first sign that something is not right with the system and therefore needs attention before a worse problem ensues. We call a mechanic and expect him to fix the issue, not just remove the light from the control board so that it doesn't bother us again! So too we really must go to the root of the medical problem rather than just easing or erasing the symptom.

That which constantly reveals itself as a series of bodily symptoms is the visible manifestation of an invisible process going on inside of us. The aim of the symptom is to show us that something is no longer in good working order and we need to investigate further and find out the cause. The symptoms we manifest are unique to each of us and offer a clue, a map to our body's hidden working system. In homeopathy, each modality of our body's reaction is listened to and interpreted in order to find the root cause in the function of the body, following the wisdom of the symptoms presented. Allopathic medicine, on the other hand, takes people as a general unit with symptoms generalised and linked to a specific disease; they cannot distinguish the form from the content. It applies enormous resources and skills to the treatment of organs and parts of the body, but never look at the individual and their unique system.

In the material world which we inhabit, it makes no sense to pit your energies against illness and death. Illness is simply a human condition which indicates a patient is no longer in 'order/harmony' at the level of their consciousness. This loss of inner balance manifests itself in the body as a symptom. Something is missing or out of balance, and therefore we are sick people or sick souls. Once people have grasped the difference between illness and symptoms their basic attitude and approach to illness becomes transformed very quickly. The symptoms are no longer seen as the enemy, but as signals from the whole that there is an issue/ an illness to sort out. The body is our friend, our dear partner in this journey of life. The symptoms that our body throws up are more intelligent than medical books or drug companies, they come out of our intimate selves and do not lie.

What we need to do when we feel unwell is to talk to our symptoms. Not to fight the illness, but to listen to it and change it back into the state of health that our minds and souls crave. We must not enter into the game of conquering symptoms. Healing is a closer approach to the whole body, a step on the way of what Jung would call the individuation process and others have called enlightenment. For once we tune in to our body's needs, we can work to supplement and grow, it is an expansion of consciousness itself.

Polarity and Unity

Polarity is a relationship between two opposite characteristics or tendencies, like the polarity of two sides of a debate, or a positive or negative electric charge. Metaphorically, it indicates something with two opposing but related qualities; it's beyond the opposites you may visualize in the plus and negative ends of a battery or magnet, it suggests opposites that are interconnected. Day and night, Yin and Yang. The very act of breathing exists as a polarity, with the breath in at one end of the pole and the breath out at the other end of the pole. This positive/negative rhythm is a constant alteration between the two poles and is the basic pattern of life, the circulation of the energy within us, commonly called meridians.

There are also two sides to our brains: the left and the right, the so-called feminine and masculine. In order to function in balance, we are called upon to use both hemispheres. Yet today's scientists are mostly only left-brain thinkers, using only their rational, reasonable, and analytically tangible functions. The basic law of polarity is not adhered to by science.

We have to understand that the irrational, the mystical, fantastical and the religious, are no more than opposite sides of the brain. At times of crisis, humans automatically switch to right brain from left brain dominance. With the right hemisphere in charge, we act calmly and competently, thanks to the timeless wisdom of the right brain, which has evolved over hundreds of thousands of years.

Unity: both poles (positive and negative) are mutually complementary, each needing the other to exist. In this way, we can see healing as a single path that leads from the polarity of veering constantly from sickness to health, to the calmness of integration and unity. Suffering can be done away with only by taking it upon oneself. Learn how to transcend the world and not to escape it, to transmute bad energy into good energy. Give up the 'I' and 'Ego' which are constantly being enforced by our society and understand that healing offers us a better road. Illness is in our nature. It is a control system which actually serves to further our evolution. If we are honest with ourselves and the healer about the issues and problems behind our symptoms, rather than the discomfort of the symptoms themselves, we may start to benefit from the advances we make in our evolution through facing and understanding our fears and our traumas. Illness makes us honest, unmasks the past.

Going back to the polarities: healing lies in sickness, just as Good lives in Evil, just as Evil lives in Good. We may not to be freed from illness, for the same reason that health actually needs it as its polar opposite. Illness is an expression of the fact that we feel sinful, guilty, fearful, etc. instead of feeling in harmony with the world around us. Rid yourself of the illusion that illness can be defeated through struggle. Illness is in our nature and we have to learn from it and make peace with it. Destroying illusions is never easy or pleasant yet always results in new freedom of movement. Listen to your inner self and enter into communication with your symptoms. Question your own views. Let your body be your guide.

PSYCHIC HEALING

There is a candle in your heart
Ready to be kindled.
There is a void in your soul
Ready to be filled.
You feel it, don't you?

Rumi

Psychic and unorthodox healing has always been a part of occult teaching, where body, mind and spirit are considered connected and therefore wanting of healing as a whole. This is in contrast to western allopathic medicine, which very clearly separates the material and emotional.

Hippocrates famously said "Physician heal thyself", meaning that any person willing to heal the sick should first of all make sure they were healthy, both physically and mentally. We will find very few physicians today who can indeed deal with their own sickness, usually consulting colleagues or other doctors. There are physicians who have treated patients while in wheelchairs. Cancer specialists who have died of cancer.

If the exhortation 'Heal Thyself' was obeyed by everyone, then both layman and doctor would benefit. Although reputable and successful healers are rare, you will find that their client base is very large, since healing is an art that is cherished.

Disease affects the whole body, the mind, the spirit. Spirit manifests in a physical body, and consequently spirit can heal the physical body. All self-healing involves a thought process, and specific thoughts influence specific illnesses.

In this psychic tradition, wrongful thoughts create illness, just as positive thoughts can reverse the condition. Such matters are entirely in the hands of the sufferer. Once the patient is cleared, the patient needs to embark on a new path of positive thought patterns. You have the power and nothing can prevent you from seeing the light and doing something about it.

In allopathic medicine illness is categorized into three causes; bacterial & viral, accidental or due to degeneration. In the field of psychic medicine, the three causes of disease are erroneous thought processes, improper living and accidents. In psychic healing, disease is the result of imbalance of the TOTAL system, that is body, mind and spirit. Disease lasts only until the imbalance is corrected, and once the balance is corrected the disease must vanish. Since spirit and mind in combination have created the body and have influence over it, it is obvious that thoughts cause disease just as they can undo it. The physical symptoms of pain and affliction are merely outer manifestations of parallel situations existing in the inner body. The job of the psychic healer is to correct the inner body and allow the outer to follow, since it will have no choice to do otherwise.

False thinking and not being able to accept the human condition, or using our energies in inappropriate ways, can cause disease, because only frustration will ensue when you can't achieve your goals. This causes damage to our systems which eventually shows up as physical disease. In such cases we can often feel stuck and fresh thinking is needed to reverse the trend and fight the desire.

No matter the nature of the decision, personal healing must be two-fold. First and foremost, one has to adopt an optimistic long-term view to overturn the effects of the disease and conquer it. Verbalizing to yourself that you have command of the disease can be done through positive affirmations and visualisations. Visualise yourself in perfect health while paying special attention to the part of the body that needs healing.[1]

The materialistic or logical thinker may think this is far-fetched, but it is an established fact that tiny electrical charges in the brain are directed by the mind. They go where they are directed to. By sending thoughts from the brain to the body you are rearranging

1 Refer to the work of Louise Hay on the emotional causes of disease and positive affirmations

the electrical molecules, purifying their positives and sending them where needed. This in turn helps to stimulates the body's defence mechanisms, thus causing physical reactions initiated by suggestion. The physical reaction then targets the diseased area mobilizing anti-toxins or natural abilities of the cells.

When dealing with pain anywhere in the body, there are two avenues; the easiest being to block the message of pain somewhere between the source and the control centre of the brain. Here we are dealing with the nerves, and at half way between source and brain we put in a road block so that the pain receptors acknowledge the roadblock and stop. The more we visualize this division the more successful we would be at blocking pain.

The second method directly addresses disease or any injured area of the body, getting to the root cause. Visualise the wound or injury in the mind's eye. Now visualise and verbalise the fact of its existence and cause. Build a protective wall around it and shut off all outgoing stimuli.

Visualise the rapid recovery of the wound or disease. Take five to ten seconds to gradually visualise it healing. By attacking the area where pain is we are killing the pain not merrily blocking it.

This method works with infection, degenerative illness, or in the case of accidental injury.

Building Your Psychic Healing Capacity

The first step is to find your spiritual centre. Learn to love yourself and others from their spiritual centre instead of from your needs and wants. Because when you understand that all is one, that everything is connected to the whole, you are freed from the necessity of passing judgment. This is the place beyond the polarities of good and evil, where there is no right/wrong, good/bad, better/worse. When you are an observer in the state of oneness, you are completely psychic. To heal a friend, you enter a state of oneness with them, then ask yourself about your friend's physical condition. Since your friend is now another part of you, another part of the whole, you already know the answer. Psychics use aura readings to determine health and the mental, emotional and psychic condition of their client.

The aura surrounds the body of living creatures and is invisible to ordinary vision. This aura is affected by ill health or disease and can change colour and shape under these circumstances. Basically, what we are saying is that the skin is not the outermost part of our bodies in space, it only surrounds the limits of the dense physical. Extending from this (for roughly two yards at its widest point and two feet beyond the head and feet) are subtle emanations deeply connected with the body and its functions. The aura is an elaborate structure of lines of force which reflect our thought processes and feelings, a subtle mirror of the whole person in a non-physical – or etheric – form. The physical health and well-being of an individual is directly linked with the condition of the aura, which is profoundly influenced by physical conditions, nutrition and hygiene. Someone who is materially starved or overfed, or poisoned with drugs or smoky air, or with insufficient or excessive exercise, will damage their physical selves as well as their aura. A person who withdraws from life and doesn't face their problems will end up with a grey, colourless aura devoid of the glow of a healthy one. When we talk about the aura here, we are referring to the physical, the emotional and the mental (mind) fields that surround the body and are connected with the workings of the parallel processes inside us.

Many psychics see aura in colour. The minimal extension of one's aura should be at least 12 inches surrounding the body Some people are walking around with incomplete auras, which leaves them open to disease, since most diseases enter through damaged auras.

Your abilities as a psychic healer depend on your willingness and ability to become at one with both client and cosmos. As a healer you can do nothing to or for someone else. You can only help them to do what they were going to do themselves anyway. If the subject is unwilling to be healed there is nothing you can do. You only become a healer to become a healer; for no other reason. You don't know what's good for someone else – your job is to help them discover their own being and their own ideas. Every person's life is their own.

Therapist Fritz Perls said: "I am not in this world to live up to your expectations and you are not in this world to live up to mine." Do not ever, as a healer, imagine that you are a doctor. Healing is only one way in which you can inspire your psychic growth. To be a healer requires very little of you, only a willingness to help.

If you want to do simple healings, learn from someone experienced, and take guidance from them. Remember that as a healer you must be grounded. The most potent and widely used techniques in healing need practise, and healing from an Alpha state.

AURA COLOUR

(If the colour is dull or washed out, it indicates low energy):

Black: Death and destruction.

Grey: Boredom/malaise. Fear and anger.

Brown: Earth colour, strong connection with earth and the physical plane. If found around the feet and legs it indicates that the person gets lots of exercise.

Green: Growth colour, change in attitude, beliefs, way of life. Positive colour may show up when the person is under the stress of major internal change.

Light apple green: a sign of psychic development.

Blue: Creativity, imagination, self-expression, feminine nature.

Dark blue: a sign of repression. When a person acts on another's ideas rather than their own.

Yellow: Intellect, changing unconscious to conscious. A halo.

Orange: Healing colour. Masculine colour. Signifies strong aura-healing power.

Pink: Intuition and instinctive knowledge about the earth, 'planetary intuition'.

Red: Emotion, warming of life, strong feelings, anger, fear, love.

Dark red: indicates repressed, troubling emotions.

Bright red: Intensity, passion.

Purple: Spiritual devotion.

Gold: Pure intuition, psychic prowess, self-knowledge. Mystics and people in state of bliss support radiant golden halos. Cleansing and healing.

Silver: Feminine colour of motion, similar to gold. Telekinesis, bending or moving objects, levitation, astral travel. Silver cord to astral body.

White: Colour of highest spiritual attainment, purification and enlightenment.

Healer/Client Relationship

When someone comes to you for a healing, they are giving consent for you to learn things about them that they might have never told their friends. They are also giving you permission to utilise your combined energies to effect change. They assume you know what you are doing and you will do whatever is needed to heal them. The healer should not act from their ego, telling the client honestly if they can't do what is needed.

Healing techniques:

» Client should sit in straight chair

» Feet flat on floor, feet and arms uncrossed

» Hands on knees, palms up

» Relax the mind

Healer:

» Stand and close your eyes, relax, clear your mind, focus full attention to client, ground yourself.

» When you are ready to heal, open your eyes (optional) place hand above the client's head and feel for heat, fullness, tingling.

» Move slowly down from the head along the neck, shoulders, arms, torso, legs, feet, sending healing energy as you go.

» If the body feels cool, it is tingling where energy is not flowing.

» Correct the flow by visualizing an orange-coloured light flowing through your hands.

» Use cosmic energy, don't ever use your own or you will be depleted.

» Cosmic energy will clear and clean, like a blood transfusion.

» You only need to will cosmic energy.

» If the aura is dense, it means there is an excess of energy in that area (blocked energy). Imagine your hands pulling it away. Pull away excess heat and dissolve it.

» Complete 5 to 6 times and then imagine a clean, clear, light golden energy flowing gently from your hands and washing over the entire body.

» Smooth the aura, rake the body down so that the aura is whole again and can protect the client from disease.

In his book, *Psychic Healing* – first published in English in 1918 – Yogi Ramacharaka put together selective healings for the reader in order to invite them to find their best method or to use combinations of several. The different techniques are all simple and can be used for self-healing, without resorting to religion or following a guru, and his book is recommended as a sound handbook of good advice.

Like all healers, he knew that energy cannot be destroyed, but it can be changed, and this is how energy healers can help. The act of healing is simply turning negative energy into positive energy. At its basis, the natural law of healing involves three processes: Nutrition, Elimination, and Breathing. Yogi Ramacharaka believed that if one followed the Hatha Yoga teachings there would be no need for healing. However, he also understood that most people would not do this, and would therefore be in need of being healed.

Like so many before him, he understood that symptoms are not what we are looking for, it is the cause. And there is only one general cause, which is malfunctioning cells, for all disease is cell disease. To facilitate healing, you'll need confidence in yourself and your healing power, and a willingness to change your habits. We all have the ability to be healers, it is not a gift for the few, but once you get results you must not become conceited, as you are only an instrument through which energy flows to where it's meant to go.

There are several paths to healing, choose the one you like or mix some of them up and find your own style of healing. Always remember, no health without Nutrition and Elimination, with elimination being the foundation. We all know what happens when we have problems in the smallest room in the house; just because we can't see what our internal plumbing is doing doesn't mean we shouldn't maintain it.

Start all healing at the stomach, as the majority of diseases start here. In terms of chakras, this is the solar plexus area of the body, the seat of our sense of personal power and self-esteem, and therefore the area of the body that needs most protection. Let's protect this area by providing it with good food and ample time for digestion. Digestion starts when the food or liquid enters your mouth, the stomach operates best when the food it receives is well chewed and sloppy like a paste. Water is also important for the body and two litres a day helps with flushing the body and the plumbing.

We also need to remember the importance of practising deep breathing, starting by just stopping at some point during our day and then breathing from our belly. You can use the Ho'oponopono prayer which you can say while breathing through the nose:

» In breath – I love you.

» Hold breath – I'm sorry

» Exhale – Please forgive me

» Hold – Thank you.

» Breathe in through the nose not through the mouth, breathe out through either.

Healers should be more than healers; they are instructors and educators. Through their closeness to the divine they become sacred healers and can help people regain their health and strength and bring them back to mother nature.

Treating
the Whole Body

Mind

Mind is the most important aspect when it comes to healing. It operates twenty-four hours a day, controlling the nourishment and operation of the physical body and the function of every organ. Repairs, replacements, physiological changes, digestion and elimination are all performed by the mind. What you tell your mind is what goes into your body. Many people become sick because of hurtful behaviour and comments directed at them which they have accepted. This leads us to the story of the boy in Egypt, sitting under a palm tree when something landed beside him:

"What are you?" the boy asked.
"I'm the Plague, and I'm heading to Baghdad to kill 5,000 people."
With that the creature left and three weeks later, he returned to the boy by the tree.
"You told me you were killing 5,000 people but I heard that 50,000 died," said the boy.
"Yes, I only killed 5,000 people, but the rest killed themselves out of fear," was the creature's response.

It is a fact that people have returned to good health with positive thoughts. When healing, always think of the person as being healed and well.

Body Cells

There is only one general cause of disease, and that is the malfunctioning of cells, for all disease is cell disease. The whole body is made of millions of cells which make up the skin, bone and tissue of the body. They select from the blood flow all that they need and reject the waste; each cell doing their own job in the overall system, protecting the body from bacteria, viruses, and fungus. Cells are like a well-run and organised city where all of them are contributing to the optimum functioning of the body. This process is controlled by the instinctive mind. The ideal is to keep the intellectual mind away from sending fearful and demoralizing thoughts to the cells. It is when the cells are overworked or malnourished that they rebel and the trouble starts. When our system is messed-up by negativity or over-exertion, illness starts to enter the body. Only with improved nutrition and proper attention will things return to normal. Science has proved that all disease is cell-based.

There are three forms of psychic healing:

- **Pranic Healing:** the sending of healing energy through the healer to the recipient.
- **Mental Healing:** control of cell function through either direct or distant healing through the instructive mind of the sick person.
- **Spiritual Healing:** the healer has use of outside energies with a greater power that pour through the patient and lift them to a higher plane.

A strong and healthy person is charged with a good supply of life force that travels to all parts of their body and surrounding aura. Depleted of this force, the person will become ill and only be restored to good health when they replenish their store of energy. The way to replace this energy is for the healer to concentrate on the area of illness with their eyes (very powerful); the passing of hands and breathing over the part of the body affected, will also aid recovery.

Find what needs to be healed, concentrate on the area with your eyes, your healing hands and your breath. That's the complete healing.

Breath can also be used to warm up healing pads so breath is quite beneficial. Rhythmic breathing helps to increase the value of mental healing, this is much the same as earlier breathing exercises, breathing through the nose:

» Sit or stand comfortably, hands on lap if possible.

» Shoulders and head relaxed.

» Inhale to the count of 6.

» Hold to the count of 3.

» Exhale to the count of 6.

» Hold to the count of 3.

Repeat as often as you can without being fatigued.

With rhythmic breathing you absorb a lot of prana or vital force. This is good for the healer as they can direct excess energy to areas of the patient's body. This way the patient is filled with prana and the diseased part is forced out of the body.

General Treatment

» Rub hands together to warm them up.

» Place the patient face down on a table with a pillow under chest.

» Move hands down the spine looking for negative energies that need healing, clear these as you go.

» Knead the back of neck and shoulders.

» Turn the patient over and work on chest arms and legs.

» Always finish with downward strokes to rake their aura clean.

General Remarks on Treatment:

The healer must at all times be governed by intuition. This will come to you; it is a healing sense that will come to you as you practise, practise, practise. Distant Healing is dependent on the mental thoughts of the healer – this can be acquired easily. One way of acquiring this ability is to say,

"I am sending you a supply of life force which will invigorate you and heal you."

How to Live Healthily

» Enjoy your body, food and exercise.
» Be comfortable with your sexuality. Express affection openly.
» Disruptive emotions need to be put in their correct place;
  constantly check these emotions and heal them.
» Let light and emotional freedom into your God-given journey.
» Give and receive without expecting return.
» Love and live for today.
» Respect nature and thank her regularly

You can also develop your psychic abilities by trying to practice maintaining a positive attitude every day. Negative thinking or excessive scepticism will impede the process or block it, but don't be discouraged – practise does make perfect and what you are trying to do is not what we were taught at school or in society. We are trying to get the energy of the head and the heart to join, to function as one. As you do this, you become healthier, happier, loving, wiser, and more open to being able to retain the healing energies.

Relaxation is very much a part of this journey; reading inspirational literature instead of tapping into the fear-mongering of mainstream media or the fool-making of popular culture and social media. Remembering our positive affirmations, and consciously replacing any frowns with smiles. Breathing deeply and being conscious of any holding in your body is also important, as we need to be vigilant in impeding bad habits from returning to our thinking, and therefore our body. If you experience discomfort, move your conscious mind to the area of your body that needs healing, tense and then relax these muscles in order to show them how to relax. Move your consciousness to your centre, to that place of radiance, love, joy peace and knowing. Now return to your body, but do it slowly.

Imagination is a vital part of our psychology. The pathways in the brain made through imagination are identical to those which occur in our thought processes in physical action – the brain does not differentiate. Athletes and artists use imagination all the time: like children, they tap into that expansive world which we all possess as children.

Psychic abilities are really soul abilities and therefore they must be trusted. "God can do no more for you than through you." The only person you can really change is yourself. Meditate and pray and use all positive thinking techniques.

When you look in the mirror, don't look for lines or something to criticise, but see the divine child. Try looking into your own eyes in the mirror and saying:
"I love you, I appreciate you, I forgive you.
Today is a new day, the past has gone.
I choose to become wiser, kinder than before.
I choose the feeling of excellence because I am unlimited in how wonderful and creative I am.
I treat others as I wish to be treated.
I respect the rights of others and respect myself."

Psychic vision needs discipline and practise, but you can build on it every day. Remember that you are the driver of your body and mind, and you can choose to drive in the right direction. In order to help you maintain your true course, you can avoid those people who divert you or try to steal your fuel, the so-called 'energy vampires', and surround yourself instead with people who share your vision. Once you start sending out love and higher waves of consciousness, it will attract the right people in, and the drive will become more and more pleasant.

Self-Healing

All that has been said before about healing others is also relevant to healing yourself. You are drawing prana (energy) from the abundant universal supply and sending it to where it is needed in or on your body. Sometimes it is a matter of only needing to balance the energy in your own body in order to set it on the right track:

» Lie flat on back, relaxed. Hands resting on the solar plexus chakra, which is located three finger-widths above the navel.
» Breathe rhythmically, and mentally direct energy to the areas of your body needing healing, imagining that you are recharging everything as you go.
» No need to use willpower, simply command energy to go where you want it to go.
» Send prana to pain areas and re-establish the circulation of energy and with that, drive out the pain.
» Breathe in and on the out-breath command that any diseased area be cleared, forced out and dispersed. Blow the out-breath over the affected area as if you are blowing the diseased area away.
» Thought-force healing is directing your mind to the part that needs healing. Tell your mind what you expect it to do and it will comply.

As stated previously, the majority of diseases start in the stomach area. So let's start there, remembering that we want to remove the cause and allow the symptom to then go away:

» Tap the stomach area with your fingers or fist and say "Stomach Mind wake up!"
» Holding your hand over your stomach say, "Now Stomach Mind I want you to wake up and attend to this organ properly, make it strong, healthy and active."
» "I want it to do this work properly, and you must see that it is so."
» "See that it digests the food properly, and nourishes the whole body. Relieve any congestion to make sure the whole organ acts in harmony with life and energy."

You do not need to repeat the exact wording of this script, but use it as an example, so that whichever organ you are healing, the healing is based around that organ. You may need to repeat this healing twice or three times daily and keep going till the healing has taken place.

Suggestive Healing

Good cheer, hope, joy, love and happiness promote growth in tissues and bones and help organs to function properly. Fear, melancholy, malice, hatred, dejection, loss of confidence and other morbid states tend to deplete the body.

Time and again people will do the same thing; they think there is something wrong with them and subsequently it manifests from nothing to something major. Turning something that is not there into a problem: it is merely a thought that has become a fear. If you want to live a long and happy life don't fall for this one. Fear is the issue that has to be dealt with. Remove the fear and you remove the disease. Replace fear with Confidence, Courage, Fearlessness, Hope.

"As a man thinketh in his heart, so he is." It's not what he says, it is what he thinks that counts. The intuitive mind will act on any suggestion passed to it, and so the aim is to restore normal thinking to those who have been thinking wrongly about their bodies. This is not hypnosis. The best results are when a patient is present with a receptive mind. First you must ascertain from your intuition if the patient wants to be healed, and if you get a negative response, you should search to see if there is a blockage that needs to be cleared. If nothing is blocking the receiving of the healing and you still get a feeling that the patient does not want healing, do not proceed, there is nothing you can do.

Once you have got the 'yes' answer – the intuition that the patient is open to healing – you can proceed.

The patient should remain relaxed, while the healer makes positive, firm suggestions/affirmations. Maintain eye contact on the area being treated. Use deep breathing, aiming the exhaled breath across the area you are healing and constantly thinking that the disease is being blown away.

Never refer to the diseased condition. Always think about the person as already healed. No negative suggestions or denials. Always positive affirmations. Remember, that it is not you who heal, it is the spirit that heals, the universal energy which is there for everybody, is what is being used.

Keep these things in mind:

» Do not become bigoted and narrow in your views.

» Do not abuse those whose opinion may differ from yours.

» Do not force your views on others, and be willing to answer questions.

» Do not abuse other health practitioners.

» Make your own work so good that people will come back to you.

» Ignore abusive members of the medical fraternity who revile the mental and spiritual healer.

» Show only passive resistance. This is man's best advice.

» Do not neglect Natural Law, proper nutrition and elimination.

» Do not go back to old habits.

» Watch out for the vampire who delights in the attention of illness and using people's energy.

» Be full of love and kindness.

» The nearer you are to the source of power the greater the power. God of Light.

» You are closer to the source of Infinite Power, which is the source of all power and it is there for all to seek.

THE WHAT AND HOW OF DOWSING

Dowsing and self-healing is easy to learn, and needs no special tool other than a pendulum. Just believe in the procedure and follow the simple instructions below. While we are not suggesting it is a substitute for medical advice, this method can be used in conjunction. Over the past years, there is a growing section of science dedicated to dowsing, with over 275 articles in peer review journals of the Association of Comprehensive Energy Psychology (ACEP) *www.energypsych.org* .

Healing yourself and others

There are Five Essentials for this to happen:

» Willingness to change

» Awareness of the condition

» Acceptance of the way you are

» Taking responsibility for what has happened

» Focusing on wellness not illness

Let go of any anger, along with any guilt or resentment which has been turned inward. Jealousy must also be removed. Fear needs to be confronted head on, without blame, and with the knowledge that faith overrides fear.

If you feel hurt, vulnerability or fear, then this must be shared. Vulnerability is a sign of strength, it's your inner child asking for support. Love is what will heal, for it is the force that moves the world.

Ten commandments of healing:

1. De-stress yourself
2. Detox your physical body
3. Nourish your immune system
4. Boost vitality with good food and supplements
5. Release negativity in your thoughts and life
6. Affirm the positive
7. Visualise health
8. Love yourself
9. Express feelings
10. Listen to the Inner Self, your intuition

The bottom line is, you are the only person who can heal you.

When you change to positive thinking, you must think of yourself first. Don't judge yourself or others, nor feel greater or lesser than others. Remove hatred and resentment from yourself and those around you, for such attitudes will cause self-destruction.

Dowsing for Health

Dowsing could be a dangerous pursuit for those with hypochondriac tendencies, since results can often be immediate. It happens that people can even diagnose cancer when still beginners. But on the other hand, beginners can also be guilty of trying too hard, and time should be taken to understand whether dowsing is a useful and compatible method for you.

One thing to remember is that dowsing is simple and there is no need to over-complicate it. Practise makes perfect. Remember that the secret of achieving accurate results from dowsing comes from integrating oneself and balancing the conscious and unconscious mind. Always remember that the subconscious is the seat of creativity and it can be a good servant but a bad master. It therefore must be properly instructed and disciplined, otherwise it tends to give the answer that it thinks the conscious self wants, or else plays up, or in certain instances gives false answers, for unconscious emotional reasons. Whenever you are about to dowse or commence a healing it is important to be sitting comfortably in a chair, or standing in a relaxed way, with your feet planted firmly on the ground. Always be careful not to cross your arms or legs, because this cuts off the energy flow.

The first thing one must do is tell the pendulum how to show the 'yes' and 'no' answer:

» Hold the chain of the pendulum between thumb and forefinger leaving about 5 cm of chain free

- » Rotate the pendulum in the clockwise direction while saying three times: "Pendulum this is my 'yes'"
- » Swing the pendulum back and forth in what will be the neutral position
- » Then ask "pendulum, please give me a 'yes'"
- » If unsuccessful, go back to the first point and go through the steps again until the pendulum responds as you want it to
- » For the 'no', rotate the pendulum anticlockwise, and say three times: "this is my 'no'"
- » Swing the pendulum back and forth in what will be the neutral position
- » Then ask "pendulum, please give me a 'no'"
- » Repeat until successful for both answers

Dowsing tips:

- » A pendulum can be any weight suspended on a chain or cord, it can be homemade or shop-bought.
- » The pendulum is an extension of your hand, attached to your own energy field.
- » Use your pendulum to increase sensitivity in detecting and gaining information.
- » Do not rely only on your own intuition but connect to your Higher Self.
- » Have faith in your ability to use the pendulum and trust the answers you get.
- » Sit at a table, elbows on table, in front of a dowsing chart if needed (see Diagram 5, page 181).
- » Relax and be at ease. Focus and check your mindset.
- » Formulate questions correctly.

» Before you start check that the 'yes' and 'no' directions you have programmed are still valid.
» If the pendulum does not respond it may be because you are tired, take a break.
» You may not be asking the right question: the answer needs to be 'yes' or 'no'.

Once you have set the pendulum you are ready to dowse. The 'yes' and the positive are the same clockwise direction; the 'no' and the negative are the same direction, that is anticlockwise.

Once you have learnt how to programme your pendulum you can now proceed to heal yourself, your family, and your friends. First up, we must remove all energy blockages from their body, mind, and soul: "Pendulum, remove all energy blockages from _____'s body, mind, and soul." Your pendulum will then rotate in the anticlockwise direction on its own, removing the negative energies. When it has finished, the pendulum will stop. Then we have to replace this energy with positive energy, calling on a power greater than ours: "God of Light, raise the energy vibration levels of _____ to the highest possible level and for the good of all." Keep repeating this total process until the pendulum is no longer indicating that there is negative energy to be removed (more detail below).

It is probably best to do this process to yourself first. If your energy levels are lower than the people you wish to heal, all that happens is you drag energy off the client and make them worse. Not the result that either of you want. These energies are sourced from the abundant energies that surround us. So let's make use of them!

Always say 'thank you' when you complete a task.

Use dowsing on yourself, others, animals, land, buildings, business, and for prosperity. All of these have a vibrational level which is what we are dowsing. Remember that the pendulum doesn't do the healing, it is only the indicator. Energy always follows thought. Everything manufactured or invented started with a thought.

Before commencing to dowse ask the questions, "May I", "Can I", "Should I". If you get a 'no' to any of these, wait and try another time.

Remember to ask "Does this person want to be healed?" If it is 'no', as hard as this sounds you must respect the answer. Ask if any blockages need to be removed. If yes, clear them and ask question again.

Always look for the cause of the problem and always dowse "For the Good of All."

It is faith not time that does the healing, so allow it to happen.

"Does this person want to be healed?"

If 'yes', do the clearing procedure as described earlier. Raise their energy vibrational levels to the highest appropriate level for the good of all by asking in that way.

Next, you need to check the client's Life Force. This must be at 100 per cent: start by asking if the life force was 100 percent at conception. If you find that the life force was not 100 per cent at conception, you can conclude that the issue is to be found in a past life.

Ask the question: "Was their life force 100 percent one past life ago? Two past lives ago...?' etc. Go back until you find where the life force was 100 percent, then bring that forward to the present day: "God of Light, please bring this person's life force from _____ past lives ago to the present day."

The What and How of Dowsing

If you find that the life force is 100 percent at conception, you then know it's not a past life issue. If the issue is in this life, you need to find the age where the disruption happened by moving forward from birth in five-yearly increments, asking "Is _____'s life force 100 per cent at age 5? At age 10..." until you find the point where it is not 100 per cent. You then go back to the point where it was last 100 per cent and ask for the life force to be brought forward to the present day, while letting the pendulum swing clockwise until is stops naturally. Then check their life force is 100 per cent at this moment.

These instructions might sound simple but you need someone to help you through the process and learn the finer details. It is easy, you've just got to know what you are doing.

"For the Good of All".

Next, we are going to check for energy vibration levels.

Setting the Programme for Your Pendulum

» First check that your pendulum is working true by checking for 'yes' and 'no'.

» Programme average energy vibration levels in your country/district by setting an energy level:

» Rotate your pendulum clockwise and say three times: "The average energy level for country/district is 30,000 units"[2]

» Let the pendulum swing in the neutral position to and fro.

» Ask: 'Pendulum is the average energy vibration level in _____ 30,000?"

» If the pendulum swings clockwise for 'yes', it has been programmed successfully.

» Checking a person's energy vibration level, which we want to be the same as, or higher than, the average energy level in the area (30,000).

» Ask the pendulum: "Is _____'s energy vibration level 30,000 or more?"

» If 'yes', then the person is healthy, but you are free to raise the unit level in your enquiry to find out what level they are at.

» If 'no', then ask using a lower number (i.e. "20,000 or more?").

» Ask questions more or less than the previous figure in order to define the energy vibration levels exactly.

---

2 Units here are the measurement I have decided upon because we have to set a figure from which to measure and compare by. I have chosen to use this instead of the Hz measurement but it means the same thing: setting 30,000 as the energy level of the Earth.

The What and How of Dowsing

Geopathic Stress
and Dowsing

As we have already mentioned, it is vital to keep in mind that everything on this earth has a vibrational level: the plants, animals, rocks, and of course, humans. We are in the position of being able to control our vibrations through our thoughts and actions, and let ourselves vibrate at a higher frequency. At this time of change, the earth is raising its vibrational levels and it is time we humans did the same as a species. Energies are important to the universe and to our lives, but it is something we have neglected in modern society. In the past, people paid attention to the energy of the land and the environment, and built where they found good energy properties. Today we build anywhere regardless of geopathic stress lines, e.g. ley lines.

It should be noted that some earth energies are beneficial while others are detrimental. These fields are known as geopathic stress or geopathic disturbances and are created by underground streams and minerals concentrations, fault lines, quarries, mine workings and other features. The relationship between the earth energies and people's well-being has become known as geopathic stress. Continuous living on these energies may result in illness and the draining of your life force. Your energy will reduce, your temperature may change, and cells become less efficient along with your power to rejuvenate yourself with regard to your immune system. Automatically your cells can physically change.

Sleeping in geopathic stress zones is particularly detrimental. While we are asleep, the body should be at rest so that it can repair itself. In a geopathic stress zone the body has to focus all its energy on combating the geopathic stress rather than focusing on regenerating and replenishment. When you sleep away from home in a non-geopathically stressed area you will notice you feel more energised.

The ancient tools that we used to check the stresses and energies in the earth are still available to us through dowsing and dowsers. You can visit land, offices and homes, looking for geopathic faults or earth's natural gridlines. Although no scientific explanation as yet has been accepted by the gatekeepers of modern science, for thousands of years people have been able to dowse for underground water wells and mineral deposits to mine.

Heal the Home, Heal the Person

When geopathic stress is corrected often the healing is accelerated. In Germany and Austria, your doctor may ask about the location of your bed and how long you have been sleeping there. This question is asked by thousands of doctors and many cancer specialist hospitals. They will recommend a geopathic survey or a visit from a geo-biologist to investigate your home before deciding on the course of therapy. To return to higher vibrational living, moving house or office is not your only option, as detrimental earth energies can be lifted and corrected from the property, nurturing and supporting your body, mind and spirit.

Firstly, I ask "Is Geopathic stress a problem for this person or family?" If I get a 'yes', I then proceed to clear the geopathic stress from the property. This can be done remotely using a rough sketch of the property, which you can draw yourself on a clean piece of paper (NB: you don't have to follow the architectural plans, you can just draw a rectangle as a representation) and using this plan I can locate the ley lines by using a pendulum in one hand and a pen in the other. When the pendulum rotates, it indicates a line of geopathic stress. With the pen I mark each stress point with a single short line by following the outline of the property which I have drawn. I then take a pen and strike through each of the marks I have made on the plan, thereby neutralising them in reality. I then do a further check for entities, curses, or bad energies in or on the property. If the pendulum indicates that there are any, I clear them remotely, so distance is not an issue.

Remove Energy Blockages

- Spin pendulum anticlockwise and say: "Please remove all energy blocks from _____, their mind, their body, their soul."
- Let pendulum swing until it stops.
- Spin pendulum clockwise and say: "Please raise the energy vibration levels of _____ to the highest appropriate level for the good of all."
- Check energy levels by saying: "Are the energy vibration levels of _____ 30,000 or more?"
- If 'no', repeat the process of the first four steps above, until 30,000 or more is achieved.

Always carry a pendulum with you and practise, practise, practise. Cup it in your hands, blow 3 breaths on it and say a small prayer internally. Then test it for the right answer by asking simple right and wrong questions.

Don't think of the answer, just let your frontal lobe rest so that you can tune in at another level. What you are doing is using the pendulum to receive answers from the Higher Self. Only call on beings that are 100 per cent from the light (if you use the dark side, it is at your peril).

Maintain only positive thoughts in your mind. Ground yourself through your feet and legs and the floor or earth beneath, then visualize a shaft of white light running from the top of your head down your spine and deep into the centre of the ground.

You must develop your ability to go to the Alpha level, or the relaxed mind. Try looking inwards, up through your forehead and placing your tongue behind the top teeth.

Remember:

» Healing power is stored in the subconscious mind and it knows the answers.

» Watch your thoughts - all frustration is due to unfulfilled desire.

» Feed the subconscious with thoughts of harmony, health, peace.

» Believe in the reality of your idea.

» All disease originates in the mind.

» There is one healing process and that is faith.

» Faith is a thought in your mind.

» Imagine the end desire and feel the reality.

» Believe in health, prosperity, peace, wealth and divine guidance.

» Pray for any loved ones who may be ill.

Dowsing for Daily/Weekly Checks

Remember to ask the question, then allow the work to happen while the pendulum is rotating, and when it stops to say 'thank you'.

» "Please remove all energy blocks from my mind, my body, my soul. Please do that now."

» "Please raise my energy vibration levels to the highest appropriate level for the good of all."

» "Please balance my immune system to the highest possible level for my best good."

» "Please raise my respiratory system to the best that it can be. For the highest good, thank you."

» "Please balance my body chemistry and pH to the most appropriate level for good health."

» "Please align all my body cells to the correct polarity so energy will flow through and energize my body."

» "Please balance and centre my whole body, including the balance of my chakras."

» "Please bring me into perfect balance and harmony with Earth energies, Universal energies, Cosmic energies and Galactic."

» "Please balance the blood flow to my brain, both hemispheres."

» "Please balance the five elements."

» "Please balance my Yin and Yang energy."

» "Please balance and raise the spirit energies of my body."

» "Please raise my life force energy to 100 per cent."

DOWSING AND RADIONICS

"God hath chosen the foolish things of this world to confound the wise and God hath chosen the weak things of the world to confound the things that are mighty; And base things of the world, and things which are despised, hath God chosen, yea, and things which are not, to bring to naught things that are. In the eyes of the world Radiesthesia is a thing of no account compared with, say, nuclear or astro-physics or atomic research, and yet... it can, when properly understood, open to us the mysteries both in this world and the world invisible. It can reveal to us the Truth in so far as our finite minds can comprehend it."

AUBREY WESTLAKE, British Society of Dowsers, speech, 1972

Spiritual Dowsing Workshop

In order to achieve the alpha state and be in touch with the Super-conscious, you should find a quiet place, close your eyes, and look through your third eye while taking three deep breaths. You can also move your eyes in a figure eight to widen peripheral vision, following an imaginary infinity symbol. Imagine white light coming through your forehead down to your feet.

Useful meditation for healing self or others:

» Sit comfortably, with your spine upright and your feet on the ground.
» Uncross your legs and arms.
» Breathe deeply in through your nose and hold for 3 seconds.
» Exhale and hold for 3 seconds.
» Repeat this three times then breathe normally and relax.
» Imagine coloured light to relieve any tension:
  "This light (or white light) through crown, down my body to my feet then through my root chakra to ground."
  (Use the name of the person you wish to receive the healing if appropriate.)
» This light penetrates into the ground and combines with golden light and comes back through feet to head.
» Open eyes.

Checking Your Pendulum for Yes/No and Negative/Positive

Dowsing is a tool you can use when you have total mental and emotional detachment. You must maintain a neutral and relaxed state, removing all emotional attachments to the outcome by taking on a 'professional detachment'.

Focus only on the question not on the answer. Let go of preconceived ideas you may have about the outcome and just keep practising with your pendulum, asking simple questions which you already know the answer to in order to check. To access the power of dowsing, we need to go to the higher self at the frequency level of Love or more. Our ego should be at absolute minimum – it needs to be bypassed so that we can form an alliance with the Higher Self.

Am I Ready to Dowse?

Ask permission of your pendulum to dowse. If the answer is 'yes', then follow by asking permission of the higher powers, asking if they have the ability to do what is to be done "For the good of all". Always remember the questions May I, Can I, Should I?

DAILY CHECK

» Tune pendulum yes/no.

» Check your energy vibration levels.

» Remove energy blocks and raise levels if you have to.

» Ask: "Am I in balance with earth energies?"

» "Please bring my total balance in line with earth energies".

» Check need for vitamins, minerals, monthly.

» Neutralise and transmute all harmful substances, heavy metals, toxins.

» Ask for chakras to be balanced and harmonised.

Do this always For the Highest Good of All

FOR DRINKING WATER

» Spin pendulum anticlockwise (negative) saying: "Please neutralise and transmute all harmful toxins and effects of this water."

» Spin clockwise, saying: "Raise the energy levels of this water to make it beneficial to drink. Thank you."

» You can also ask the question:
"Is this food/drink good for me?"

DOWSING FOR WATER QUALITY

A useful reference tool for checking water quality is the Mager Rossette Colour Wheel[*3] , which you can find and print off from the internet. Hold the colour chart between thumb and first finger,

---

3 The Mager Rossette Colour Wheel can be easily found on the internet

pointed at colour/water quality you want to check and use pendulum in other hand. You can improve your skills in this if you dowse first using water samples. It's best to work alone so that you are not influenced by others.

Violet Best spring water

Blue Normal drinking water

Red High Iron

Grey Polluted water, carrying lead

Black Geopathic stress adversely affecting health

White Reputed healing springs, where silver is diluted in water

Green Mineralised, e.g. copper

Yellow Hard water, e.g. magnesium

ALLERGIES

» Spin pendulum anticlockwise (negative) saying: "Go back in time and change the DNA to enhance the immune system. Neutralise effects of offending food or item upon this person."

» Check if issue is resolved with the pendulum using yes/no answers.

FOR UNHELPFUL, LIMITING THOUGHT PATTERNS OR SELF-DESTRUCTIVE PROGRAMMES

» Spin pendulum anticlockwise (negative) saying:
"Please clear and remove all self-destructive programmes and transmute their energy into positive loving energy. Thank you."

FOR THE NEGATIVE EFFECTS OF POLLUTANTS SUCH AS TV MEDIA MASS CONSCIOUSNESS, COMPUTER GAMES

» Spin pendulum anticlockwise (negative) saying:
   "Please scramble, deactivate and adjust their frequencies into a pure thought form."

CHECKING YOUR ENERGY VIBRATION LEVELS

» Remove all energy blocks by allowing the pendulum to spin anti-clockwise (negative rotation), while saying:
   "Please remove all blockages from this person's body, mind, soul".

» Wait for pendulum to stop.

» Then rotate pendulum clockwise (positive), saying:
   "Please raise the energy vibration levels of _____ to the highest appropriate level, for the good of all."

» Check if person is in balance with earth.

» Raise to the highest appropriate level, and for the good of all.

CHECKING FOR PSYCHIC CORDS

» Ask the pendulum to confirm if there are any psychic cords attached to body, mind or soul.

» If 'yes', move your hand from the top of your head down towards your feet in a slicing motion, as if cutting all cords in its path.

» Check with pendulum once again to see if you have been successful.

CHECKING FOR NEGATIVE SPIRITS

These are spirits that have not passed to the other side after the death of their material bodies. They attach themselves to like-minded people still alive, and through them carry on their previous bad habits, addictions, negative behaviours, etc. In order to maintain physical and mental health, we need to check and remove negative energies, entities and non-beneficial spirits:

» Ask if there are any negative energies, entities or non-beneficial spirits attached to the body, mind or soul.

» If 'yes', clarify which type, i.e. "Is it negative energies?" "Is it non-beneficial spirits?" etc.

» We have to deal with each of these categories separately, helping them to cross over onto the other side.

» Allow the pendulum to rotate, saying:
"Negative energies/entities/non-beneficial spirit please move over to the other side, re-join your friends and family, you will be happy there."

» When the pendulum stops of its own accord, this indicates that the spirits have left the person.

Radionics

Radionics is the theory that every life form on this planet exists in the electro-magnetic field of the earth, held between the two poles. Human beings, along with animals and the insect and plant kingdoms, are all part of this field, formed of waves and vibrations, that makes up the universe. Just as we are part of the whole, we also have our own individual electro-magnetic field which, if sufficiently distorted, will eventually lead to disease.

These waves and vibrations affect all living creatures and can have beneficial effects, while others can be harmful and all living things are affected by them. Everything vibrates at its own particular frequency and even on the level of the body itself, each organ and part of the body has its own separate vibrational level which must be maintained for health.

Each disease or harmful substance has its own vibration in the body, as well as any physical, emotional and spiritual traumas or imbalances. Remedies too, have their own particular frequency or vibration rate, and this is what homeopaths use when they prescribe a remedy; relying on the vibration of the diluted substance to stimulate the energy of the Vital Force in the patient to promote balance and healing.

As a healing art, radionics encompasses physics, para-physics, science and religion. The success of radionics is intent, as the intention to heal is the foundation of any healing process. The healing is only as good as the healer, and that healer must be emotionally removed from the process. Do the work and move on to the next issue. Radionics does not profess to be a medical diagnosis, prescription of a remedy or cure. It is a means of identifying and assessing the underlying causes. All radionics is practised recognising that our thoughts create our environment. Body is a product of mind, and we are in control of what we put into our mind, with bad thoughts being particularly powerful or 'thrice cursed' by harming the thinker, doing injury to their mental body and harming mankind and the whole mental atmosphere. Radionics can detect not only current imbalances but also future and potential fields. Long before a problem will manifest as a physical symptom it will show up as an energy imbalance.

Radionics is not a new healing concept. According to Dr Aubrey Westlake, former Chairman of the British Society of Dowsers, the earliest European reference to it was in A.D. 1240, and the first reference in England was in 1638 in a book written in Latin by Robert Fludd. The scope of dowsing at that time was almost entirely limited to water and mineral ore dowsing. The premise for the art of dowsing is based on the discovery that all matter radiates energy and that everything has a unique vibration of its own and therefore all radiation emitted can be detected and measured. Correctly applied radionics can detect, then heal disease working on 'matter = energy'.

Remember that radionics can be used to produce negative, destructive energies if used in the wrong way. It is advisable to keep away from dark energies, or any need for revenge or getting even, as destructive impulses and thoughts return to the sender.

Albert Adams stated he worked on a scale of one to one hundred in order to find a measurement system for detecting energy levels. He found that the energy levels of diseases actually differ: for example, Syphilis had a rate of 55, Gonorrhoea was 52, whereas TB was 42 on the scale. So what did he mean by a rate of vibration? It refers to the energy vibration levels of everything, for everything has a rate. It comes down to the skill of the operator (dowser) to find the frequencies that are not right (illness), and alter them back to the correct frequencies. Operators know that the rate is based on the infinite number Pi. You will find a Pi rate in a cabbage, a person, income tax: basically, everything that exists in the universe.

What I am going to describe here is paper radionics, which is based on a special geometric rosette design – or graphic – whereby the correct rate, or a prepared remedy, is placed on one of the outside circles and the person or place where the healing is to be directed, is placed in the centre (see Diagram 6, page 183). This healing relies on the ability of the operator to be capable of sending the required healing. To be able to facilitate this you should have a very good understanding of dowsing, searching for information with the help of the pendulum. Let it be remembered that neither the pendulum nor the dowser seek out the problem nor solve the issue. It is a higher energy than a human one that is in play here – it is Universal Energy.

To know the true rate of something is to have power over it. The radionicist/dowser must know their inner self because this is where the information is coming from. Using the pendulum you look for the problem, analyse what may be needed to clear the situation, find the remedy or rate and put them on the specifically designed graphic (the 'rosette' found in Diagram 6), then place the person's name in the very centre, and the healing will start. Allow yourself to sink into the required trance in order to utilize the power of the earth. Radionics can be used to send instant healing to anywhere or anyone in the world or universe. You simply use the correct rate for what you are wanting to heal, place the person or object that you are healing in the centre. Send your thoughts and thank the higher self. Simple.

Dowsing
for a Rate

We are now using a numerical healing source in order to find the correct rate. Numbers are a form of energy (kinesthetic) so the rate of everything can be represented by a number. We do not use science to diagnose, we simply ask the question and let the pendulum tell us the answer. Under no circumstances should we tell the pendulum the answer, or else our dowsing will suffer and give incorrect information. By using the pendulum, we can find the healing rate.

Suppose we have found that something/someone is not right and we need a rate to fix the problem. Firstly, we ask the pendulum how many numbers are needed for the rate, e.g. 4 numbers may be required. We therefore ask: 'What is the first number?'. To make this process easier, we can ask: 'Is the first number 5 or more?' If it's less, you count backwards (e.g. 4, 3, 2, 1, 0) and if it's more, you simply count from 5 until 9. We can then ask what the second, third and fourth numbers are, using the same process. Let us say that after this process, we end up with a rate of 2, 6, 4, 9 for the problem to be fixed. We would then write this number down on a piece of paper and place it on one of the outside circles of the rosette, then add the name of the person or thing that needs correcting in the central circle.

You can also look up a rate in a book or online, where you will find resources available for free.[4] Let's say you are healing asthma: you

---

4   SCRIBD has a number of Radionics Rates books available for a small monthly subscription fee. Also see: *http://www.royalrife.com/rates.pdf*

look the rate up and there are several rates for asthma. Your next step would be to use your pendulum and dowse for which rate is the most appropriate for the healing, e.g. Royal Rife rates for osteoarthritis; 10800, 521523, 220192, 211015, 03033, 27490. Put the number on an outside circle of the rosette, and the person's name in the centre and let the healing start.

Radionics and Radiesthesia

Radiesthesia is the term for radionics that deals with the area of medicine. It is when we search for energy waves and vibrations in the universe that are connected with health and healing. Remember, everything in the universe has a wave length or vibration.

Some tips on getting results from your pendulum:

1. Ask simple clear questions that only require a yes/no answer.
2. Only use one question in a sentence at a time.
3. Always use positive questions, 'Is this?' not 'Isn't this?'
4. Be sincere, not curious.
5. Never hurt anyone with your questions. Please avoid any ill-intent, as it will come back to bite you badly.
6. Be careful with the way you use the pendulum when gambling.
7. It is advisable to vary your questions when practising and practising is what you have to do.

Radionics can broadcast healing frequencies by altering the electro-magnetic field of the person or object it is sending the healing to. It is the focus and the intent of the operator that makes the success of the healing, and in that way, radionic healing is similar to hands on healing, both send healing through waves to where they are to go. When radionic healing is set up on the rosette as described above, it can continuously send healings to the target. We have included eleven radionic combinations for common conditions at the end of this book (see Diagrams 7–17, pages 185–205). Although the best healings happen with the pendulum indicating that the healing is finished, which usually takes 20 sec to 3 min. At this point, it is best to remove the rate and set the healing up again to be sent to the target at a later time.

Combining the techniques of both radionics and hand-healing makes for a good understanding of both, increasing your healing ability.

Radionics is a healing and diagnosis performed at a distance by the operator using healing cards and/or numbered healing rates which have been calculated by the operator. This is done by diagnosing the present energy vibration rate and if it has to be adjusted, to then set up a rate to send to the person or object needing the healing. Radionics understands that everybody's vibrations are as unique as their fingerprints. When illness, injury, infection, stress, pollution, malnutrition, poor hygiene, cause our usual patterns to become unbalanced, then radionics can return them to the right frequencies. Radionics is used with animals, land and crops, and is complementary to homeopathic remedies, acupuncture and reiki. It treats any illness through the auric field and the effectiveness of the treatment is limited only to the ability of the operator.

What can be done with Radionics?

» Assess health of others
» Find cause of the problem
» Select healing remedy
» Vibrational requirements for healing
» Is this food good for you?
» Analyse soil, plants, pets and crops
» Find geopathic stress or other harmful energies in house, office or farm

FAITH IS
THE OPPOSITE
OF FEAR

"But He was wounded for our transgressions,
He was bruised for our iniquities;

The chastisement for our peace was upon Him,
And by His stripes, we are healed."

Isaiah 53:5

Granville Oral Roberts, an American Charismatic Christian televangelist, said that you must have faith in God for your own healing. He reminded us that Jesus suffered 38 stripes, and that doctors have classified 38 major diseases. Jesus has healing stripes for every disease. We could add that one must have faith in whatever path of healing one chooses to follow, stepping onto the healing path to heal.

Healing Begins Within

You may have noticed and asked yourself the question, why are human beings dominated by fear? The answer is simply that they are not using their faith because they are out of tune with God. When we come to this life, many of us forget that we are a Divine spark, that we are one with God. We experience trauma, start thinking that we are alone, and allow fear to enter our hearts.

A person's biggest troubles are within, people are condemned by their own negativity, which means that faith alone will not work. And without faith the soul is no match for the gruelling grind of life. We have to understand that God is the only healer. While doctors – both allopathic and homeopathic – can perform great work, they are in actual fact only assisting nature.

When you feel the power of healing surging through your body in answer to faith prayer, leave aside your old ways and believe that a higher power is with you on every step of your new journey. Undo all the harm that wrong thinking and doing has inflicted on you. And change your outlook to a sunny disposition.

Affirmations
for Healing

Healing is a big part of our spiritual journey. The corporatisation of health and legislation have stolen our natural inheritance from us: our connection to the earth, the healing herbs and minerals we used to rely on, the daily worship of eating well and loving nature. We have been taught that time is a commodity, that diseases can be cured by a pill, and then we have been sent back to work work work. Perhaps healing is simply an awakening to who we truly are.

Don't wait for a crisis to make a change

» Release the past

» Don't try to please everyone

» Discover what gives you joy and zest

» Don't wait for a crisis to change your life

» Be at peace with yourself

» Don't judge a person by their worst qualities but by their best qualities

» Do not cancel people out because they don't fit your frame of things

» Never be a captive of your fears

Asking the Divine for Psychic Protection

While using the pendulum to dowse, you can call on God for constant help:

» Ask the Lord of Light to shield your self, your house, your car, your workplace with pure golden light.

» Ask the Lord of Light to heal every cell of your body and fill in holes in your aura with pure golden light.

» Ask the Lord of Light to remove all dark energies from your body, mind, soul, and aura.

» Locate any lost soul parts. Ask to cleanse, heal and integrate them back to your body, mind, soul.

» Ask to remove any energies that are not yours from your body, mind and soul, and to protect yourself, your family and friends from darker energies.

Contacting God (Praying)

In Spiritual Healing vital energy is imparted to the system from without. To invoke this energy, there are ways to open your system to its power:

» You must be in a state of relaxation to receive an influx of spiritual energy.

» Take energy from the top of your head down to your toes.

» Breathe slowly and regularly.

» Repeat this for two days.

» On the third day, breathe while saying internally: "I am Power", "I am Strong","I am Health", "I am Well" and maintain this exercise for five minutes.

» Send out a mental call for help and it will come, but you must make sure you are in good health, maintaining an attitude of kindness, and with your mind in a receptive/sympathetic mood.

» Place one hand either over your third eye or on the solar plexus, and ask divine spirit to come in and help.

In Spiritual Healing vital energy is imparted to the system from without, and there is magnetic energy contained in every living body, waiting for the healing to come. When our health is optimised, disease is depleted. The vital healing energy fills the nerve centres and adds new life to the whole body as these nerve centres become stimulated, enabling various functions of the body to be invigorated and allow the patient to heal.

Cosmic Power pervades the universe, and we draw on it. The more we draw, the faster the healing.

Sending Healing to Someone

» Open your left hand

» Blow a cool breath onto the palm three times, saying:
"This is the Antidote to the Problem"

» Lay the left hand on the forehead of the patient, saying:
"All darkness shall be gone"

» Take your right hand and blow warm air onto the palm three
times

» Then place your palm on the patient's forehead, saying:
"This breath comes from God and shall heal all the damage that
was done"

Healing from a Distance

As above (imagine your hand on the patient's forehead)

» "Every day I feel healing happen. Every day in hypnosis."

» "I send healing energies of white light to _____ until completely
healed."

Faith is the Opposite of Hear

Healing With Your Fingers

To prepare for this way of healing, which is very effective and simple, you must find the polarity of the first and second finger of the hand that is not your pendulum hand.

» Hold your pendulum in your normal dowsing hand. Let's say in this case it is your right hand. If you are left-handed, just do the following procedure with the opposite hand:

» Hold your pendulum in right hand and with your left hand, fingers spread, place your hand on the table.

» With no thoughts at all in your mind, swing the pendulum in the neutral to and fro, then hold the pendulum in front of the first finger and wait for the pendulum to indicate what polarity it is.

» It will spin anticlockwise for negative polarity or clockwise for positive polarity.

» Now change to the second finger and if the test is true it will spin in the opposite direction to the first finger.

For this task, we are only interested in the first and second finger, but if you check the third finger it will be the same as the first. The fourth finger will be the same as the second finger. Try the thumb and it will not register at all. Our body is electrically charged like a torch battery, + positive and – negative.

Now you are ready to heal using the first two fingers of your hand and the pendulum. It must be stated that the pendulum does not do the healing. It shows you where the problem is and how long the healing will take. You can do the healing on the person or yourself directly or a distant healing by using a drawing of the human form on paper (see Diagrams 1 and 2 on page 179). Just scan the body with your free hand, holding a pencil as a pointer and with the pendulum swinging in neutral position. When the pendulum swings in the negative direction anticlockwise, that is where the trouble is.

Now we start the healing. Firstly, we use the negative polarity finger and place it on the area that needs the healing. Now this is where you can cheat; spin the pendulum in the negative (anticlockwise) and say "Please remove all unwanted energy from here now", then let the pendulum swing naturally till it stops. Then change your finger to the positive polarity finger, spin the pendulum in the clock-wise direction and say "Please raise the energy vibration level to the highest appropriate level, and for the good of all". Let the pendulum run itself down.

Now repeat the process again until the point where the pendulum ceases to spin when you ask to take unwanted energy away. At this point, the healing has been effective, although you may have to repeat the total process three or four times until total relief is found.

Healing Through Meridians

On page 180 you will find a diagram of the body (front and back) with the meridian points for the main organs. In Ancient Chinese medicine, the meridians in the body carry Qi or life force through special channels that connect the various organs and functions. These meridians are designed to work together so that the body, mind, and spirit work as an organic whole. A meridian is a point through which life energy flows, and this is where the acupuncturist would position a needle in order to promote healing or activation of a particular organ function. In this case, we shall be using our fingers in the same was as described above, drawing out the negative energy with the negative finger, and healing energy with the positive finger. Don't forget that it may take more than one time to have effect – keep checking with the negative finger, and if the pendulum is still swinging anticlockwise, you know that you need to continue with the procedure until the pendulum stops completely when your negative finger is on the chosen meridian. You can also check the next day to make sure that the issue has been resolved.

Healing the Chakras and the Energetic Flow

When we are performing healing on someone from a distance, we can do this by running through each of the chakras of the person, using a drawing of the outline of a body which represents the person needing to be healed. Working with the pendulum, as above, we move down the seven chakras. Each chakra has a vibration of its own, as does each organ of a person's body, and it is the chakra's job to supply the energy to the organs under its sphere of influence. Let's give a short description of each chakra and how it works, working from the head down to the toes, from the seventh to the first chakra:

7 **Crown Chakra** – in touch with the heavens above us, this is the seat of wisdom. The crown chakra is linked to every other chakra and so it affects all our organs too, but also our brain and nervous system. Considered the chakra of enlightenment, it represents our connection to our spiritual sense and purpose. Those with a blocked crown chakra may seem narrow-minded, sceptical, or stubborn. When this chakra is open, it is thought to help keep all the other chakras open, and to bring the person bliss and enlightenment. The colour associated with the crown chakra is violet, and this chakra has the highest vibrational energy and is associated with inner searching and spiritual quest. This chakra is linked to the pineal gland and operates best when body, mind and soul are balanced, that is, having the trinity of the body, mind and soul in line.

Third Eye Chakra – the seat of the all-important guide of intuition and imagination. Blockages can manifest as headaches, issues with sight or concentration, and hearing problems. People who are deaf to others and only hear their own opinions, who are not in touch with their intuition, may have a block. The colour associated with the sixth or third eye chakra is indigo blue, and its position in the middle of the forehead, slightly above the eyes. Its energy is drawn from the pituitary and pineal gland. This is the intuitive chakra and is used in developing people's psychic centres during the art of meditation. If illness happens through the third eye it is highly likely the person is holding or trying to avoid solving an issue or problem by not dealing with it.

Throat Chakra – our means of communication and verbal expression. Voice and throat problems as well as any problems with everything surrounding that area, such as the glands, the teeth, gums, and mouth, can indicate a blockage. Blocks or misalignment can also be seen through dominating conversations, gossiping, speaking without thinking, and having trouble speaking your mind. Alignment and balance in this chakra brings confidence and compassion in our speech. The fifth chakra is associated with the colour sky blue. Because the throat deals with thyroid and parathyroid glands it is also responsible for our bone structure. It is important in communication and dysfunction in this chakra leads to poor communication and self-expression. Songs and flowing words come from a fully functioning throat chakra.

The lower four chakras represent earthy energies. Earth, Water, Fire, and Air. The top three represent the etheric and higher spiritual energies.

4 **Heart Chakra** – the heart is all important; the seat of love and joy. When this chakra is blocked or joy and love are denied, the heart suffers, asthma can develop, and there can be weight issues. It's the middle of the seven chakras, so it bridges the gap between our upper and lower chakras, and it also represents our ability to love and connect to others. Since many of our actions come from the heart, a tell-tale sign of blockages can be putting others first, to the detriment of oneself, making us feel lonely, insecure, and isolated. The heart chakra is associated with the colour green, and an open heart chakra is an expression of love to yourself and others. The highest form of spiritual love is unconditional love for others. Many people experience problems with developing inner love and little do they know that this leads to heart disease. The heart chakra is one that should be studied in more depth as it is tied to cancer, strokes and heart attacks.

3 **Solar Plexus Chakra** – this is located three finger widths above the belly button and is the seat of our self-confidence and our sense of 'I' and personal power. Blockages in the third chakra are often experienced through digestive issues like ulcers, heartburn, eating disorders, diabetes and indigestion. The colour associated with the solar plexus chakra is yellow. This can be a problem area as many people seem to leave themselves open to attack by having an open solar plexus chakra, meaning that they create an environment where other people's negative energies tend to enter your body and get stuck. Sometimes these energies take so long to leave that there is a build-up in this area that leads to illness. Blockage of the solar-plexus chakra can lead to anger, rage and abuse. If this chakra is not cleared the person becomes dominant and controlling.

2 **Sacral Chakra** – not surprisingly, this is the seat of our creativity, sexuality and pleasure. Issues with this chakra can manifest in problems with the nearby organs, like urinary tract infections, lower back pain, impotency, large and small intestines, appendicitis. Emotionally, this chakra is connected to our feelings of self-worth, and even more specifically, our self-worth around pleasure, sexuality, and creativity. The colour associated with the sacral chakra is orange.

1 **The Base Chakra**, also known as the Root Chakra, indicates how strongly we are connected to the earth. Here is where we develop our sense of being grounded and the ability to make good decisions. It is located at the very base of our physical body, between the genitals and the anus, and is the seat of our stability and physical identity. A blocked root chakra can manifest as physical issues like arthritis, constipation, and bladder or colon problems; or emotionally through feeling insecure about finances or our basic needs and wellbeing. Haemorrhoids and other anal problems are also associated with a blocked base chakra. This chakra controls the elimination of wastes so if it is not functioning properly there is a build-up of waste in the body. The associated colour is red and the creative energies can be channelled through the base chakra either as creative thoughts or reproduction of the species. When this chakra is in alignment and open, we will feel grounded and secure, both physically and emotionally.

Detecting Illness and Healing

You can detect future diseases that are developing in humans, animals, and plants by dowsing.

Ask your pendulum these questions.

1. Do I/they have a health problem?
2. Is it located in the physical body?
3. Is it in the mind?
4. Is it in the auric field?

Once we have ascertained the answers to these questions, we need to know which chakra the disease is related to. Start from the base chakra and dowse to see which chakra area needs clearing:

Chakra	Associated Gland	Body Area
1. Base/root	Adrenals	Spinal column, Kidneys
2. Sacral	Gonads	Reproductive organs
3. Solar Plexus	Pancreas	Stomach, Liver, Gallbladder, Nerves
4. Heart	Thymus	Heart, Blood, Vagus nerve, Circulatory system
5. Throat	Thyroid	Bronchia, vocal apparatus, Lungs, Alimentary canal
6. Third Eye	Pituitary	Lower Brain, Left eye, Ears, Nose, Nervous system
7. Crown	Pineal	Upper Brain, Right Eye.

The major organs that can be checked by dowsing through the chakras are: Heart, Lungs, Right and Left Kidney, Brain, Hands and Legs.

The seven chakras are the main chakras or power sources of the body, and we can dowse each chakra either by holding the pendulum over the chakra in its position on the body, or by holding the pendulum at your side and locating each chakra with your free hand, laying your hand on top of the chakra and seeing which way the pendulum spins in response. So, if your pendulum rotates anticlockwise on the Solar plexus chakra we know that we have a problem with either the stomach, the liver, the gallbladder or the nervous system. Best to have these written down somewhere, or a dowser's chart (Diagram 5, page 181) so that you can then use this in conjunction with your pendulum to specify which organ or body part needs healing by working through the list and asking.

The chakras (seen as spinning wheels of energy inside us which regulate our bodily functions), when working as they should, provide the body with energy. We must understand that our chakras operate on the emotions that we create. If our energies are not good there will be a lowering of performance by the chakras. You must start to understand that to have a healthy body and mind, you have to love yourself and others unconditionally. Tell yourself several times a day that this is possible. Love is the source of all healing. Use the power of meditation, visualization, prayers and affirmations to bring this message home. Stay in the now, making sure you are grounded.

Staying in touch with your healing energies

To begin healing work, get in touch with your own healing energies.
Fully in touch with white light. Bring it down through your core
to your sacral chakra, saying: "I open my crown, third eye, throat,
heart, to unconditional love, joy, compassion, to divine healing."

» Open all your chakras front and back with white light. Fill them
with white light.

» Then fill the aura around you with white light.

» Now fill the house, the town/city, country, then universe, with white
light.

» Imagine the person you want to heal is within your aura. Now
send white light down their crown chakra.

» Imagine golden or silver hands above their head.

» Concentrate on the person and send universal prayer that they
be totally healed.

» Gently let the person disappear and then direct attention to the
next person.

» When finished, bring your attention back to the room.

» Gently let the light or energy disappear, then cancel.

Before you start, take at least three deep breaths and relax while
you are working.

Dowsing Yourself and Others

To dowse yourself or conduct a distant healing, draw an outline sketch of what or who you are healing (for the human body, you use the diagrams on page 179) and include the chakra system either on paper or in your imagination.

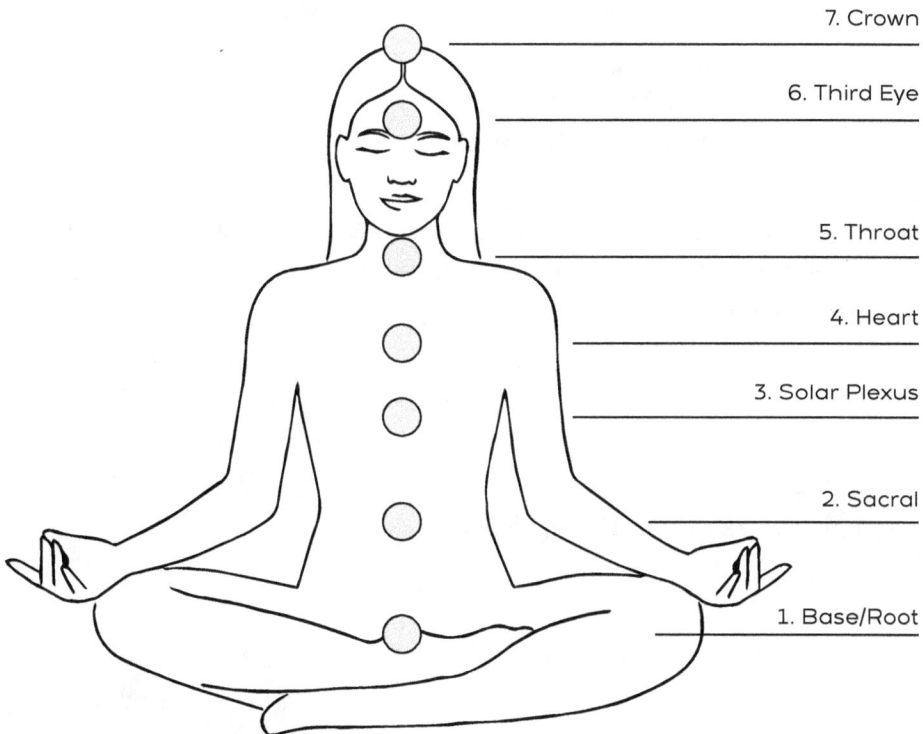

7. Crown

6. Third Eye

5. Throat

4. Heart

3. Solar Plexus

2. Sacral

1. Base/Root

» Hold your pendulum over each chakra in turn and if any show a negative, clear the chakra by spinning the pendulum anticlockwise while saying, "Pendulum please remove all energy blocks from the _____ chakra now."

» When the pendulum stops, spin the pendulum in the clockwise motion and say: "Raise the energy vibrational levels of the _____ chakra to the highest possible level and FOR THE GOOD OF ALL"

» Keep repeating (both the removing and raising processes) till your pendulum no longer swings anticlockwise, meaning there is no more negative energy to remove at that time. The healing is complete for this session.

These are some points on how chakras can keep you healthy or how illness can occur within the imbalance of the body. Each chakra is responsible for its own part of the body, and when the chakra is not working as it should, you can find out which organ you need to heal, sometimes long before the doctor picks up what's wrong. Yes, there are doctors out there that use a pendulum; what they – and we – are looking for is an uninhibited flow of energy through the whole body. If this is not happening then we remove the blockage and get the energy flowing again. When it comes to the flow of energy, we don't just look at the physical body we also look at the etheric field, which is basically your auric field that surrounds the physical body. Many illnesses that enter the body come through the etheric field. Something happens in the outside reality and this then enters the body through a weak area of the auric field.

Key points:

» Chakras bring in energy and distribute it to the body.

» It is your emotions that affect the flow of energy.

» A blockage in any chakra over a long period of time can cause illness.

» Be especially wary of blockages in the heart chakra, as this can lead to major problems.

» Meditation is a good way of unblocking and clearing chakras.

» The root chakra holds lots of energy to distribute throughout the body.

» Physical problems can be related to unresolved stress.

» Repeating affirmations is the best way to heal negative thoughts about yourself and others.

Healing Yourself and Your Surroundings

Many times, the root of illness lies not in the body or the soul, but in the mind. The mind of the client may be programmed for self-punishment or over-protection because of past traumas that may have occurred when they were too young to remember, or have been locked behind a wall of forgetting in order to ease their burden. Keep this in mind and dowse the body and psyche for traumas that effect health.

If you have asked the pendulum the question 'Does this client want to heal?' and received a positive answer, you then have to ask yourself if you come across conditions which do not improve while dowsing: "Why does this client's body not heal?"; "What does this client need to know to heal themselves?". You need to find the reason that the client's healing has been blocked; which must be due to external influences (negative energies, entities, non-beneficial spirits).

All of us have to learn to deal with and resolve disharmony in the body, mind and soul by understanding our emotions and trying to solve any blockages. A healer's job is to help others heal by unblocking stuck energies and so enabling the healing. We can open a door in the client for them to understand themselves better and to take steps towards health. We must remind them of the three steps they can take towards empowerment:

Faith is the Opposite of Hear

- Take responsibility for your health. Two thirds of ailments clear themselves, given time. You and nature have the combined power to heal yourself. Remember that the doctor is a facilitator of healing, not the healer. No healing is done until the client allows it to happen.

- Staying healthy and dealing with the sickness. Always keep in mind that the food you eat and how you eat it is vitally important. The moment food goes in your mouth your stomach is preparing itself to receive it, so masticate properly in your mouth before releasing it to your stomach. Dowsing can help you select the type of foods you should be eating if intolerances are an issue. Once you understand that you are responsible for your health, look for a regime you are comfortable with and that you are prepared to stand by with family and friends.

- Decide how far you want to go with your self-healing. How much pain and agony will you stand before calling a doctor? In no situation do we want to get stubborn and not seek medical help. You just need to develop self-knowledge which will allow you to set your own borders and understand what you can do alone, and what you need help with. Healing goes beyond the physical body, it involves psychic and healing energies, astral planes, chakras, meridians, mind, ego, soul, etc. Dowsers do not diagnose or treat illness; they channel the Higher Energy through to the client for them to use. Once the clients allow themselves to self-heal the healing can take place.

Negative Energies

At the very least, we must be constantly careful as to where we are investing our time, and which establishments we frequent. We want to work and live in places of positive energy, not ones where addiction, greed or submission of self is required.

Experienced dowsers can locate 'geopathic force lines' or 'ley lines' across the land, and even find offshoots from the main streams of energies (known as whorls), which manifest in negative or positive nodes. Positive nodes would be the places that most animals might seek when giving birth, although it should be noted that cats – ever contrary – like to sleep in the negative nodes. Such negative nodes are avoided in many traditional cultures (take the art of Feng Shui) when it comes to building their homes, fearing the unhealthy effects of living there. In terms of archaeology, dowsing can be useful in identifying the positive nodes in order to locate the sacred buildings and stone circles built by our ancestors.

We also have to remember that the spirit world is ever present, but that it is us who must reach out to them. The first thing you have to do if you feel the presence of darkness and deception in your life is to ask for help:

» Ask if there is any reason not to do this and if you are able to do this.

» Ask to remove all curses, hexes and spells put on a person, place or thing: hold the pendulum and let it rotate anticlockwise until it stops. Then replace the energy you have removed with love, by letting the pendulum rotate clockwise. In this way, you can transfer any non-beneficial thought forms from a person, place or thing and transform them into pure love.

Remember that energy is imprinted on matter. Bad things happen on the land and the imprint stays there until someone knows how to remove it. This is what we call geopathic stress. When assessing the state of a place or building, ask if there are any problems with geopathic stress and identity where it lies so that you can focus the healing there. Neutralise all geopathic stress by allowing the pendulum to swing anticlockwise until it stops naturally, and then turning the energies into love with the clockwise swing as explained previously in the Dowsing and Radionics chapter, page 101.

Everything has a spirit, including rocks and inanimate objects. All the human emotions such as love, greed, etc also have spirit. To neutralise them say: "I take all negative energies, entities and non-beneficial spirits, greed, grief, sadness, neutralise them and turn them into pure love."

Clearing Negative Influences

This accomplishes two important functions: troubled humans who have been afflicted with bad spirits have them cleared, allowing normal function of their freewill, and spirits are sent to a place where they can evolve spiritually.

This is rescue work, so we must always be gentle, considerate and non-judgemental. The spirits themselves are in need of guidance and instruction: send them to the other side and tell them their deceased family and friends are waiting for them. Reassure them that they will be fine once they cross over.

We want to enable the person to achieve harmony and peace of mind so that they have power over those that create disharmony. We want their personal relationships, finance, health, work and home environment all to exist in harmony with each other. Harmony in a person's life strengthens personal relationships, it even establishes better relationships between adversaries.

When working to clear the bad spirits from a person's body, mind or soul, we must maintain an intention:

"I visualize you standing in a circle of your family and friends. There is joy in your hearts, a smile on your lips. There is compassion and trust for one another. There is an all-embracing love, there is complete harmony. There is peace of mind knowing all is well with this wonderful group of people. All are truly grateful and thankful for this wonderful feeling."

The above can be as powerful as any exorcism. It can be beneficial also to wider communities, nations, or even the whole of humanity, imagining them in a heart circle of light. Once the bad spirits have cleared, the turnaround can happen in hours.

In world affairs as well as personal affairs, harmony is the key.

"This is the way of peace,
Overcome evil with good,
Falsehood with truth and hatred with love."

The Golden Rule – "Do unto others as you would have them do unto you" – would do as well.

Please do not take or say these intentions lightly or dismiss them as mere religious concepts that are of no practical help. They are the laws governing human conduct, which apply as rigidly as the laws of gravity. What some people call Natural Law, the law that must govern human actions and relations. When we disregard these laws in any walk of life, chaos results.

Through a return to these laws and an obedience to them, this frightened, war-weary world of ours could enter into a period of peace and richness beyond our fondest dreams for this life.

A healer taps the source of Healing Power and directs the healing to the person who needs it. This can be sent to one person or many people at a time. For example, when dealing with trauma that gets passed on from generation to generation one can heal that trauma not only from the person who experiences it at that moment in time, but also from the whole lineage across time and space, past, present and future. By doing so one can erase it from the fabric of the universe.

Using a pendulum, one can determine the state of health of each person, expressed in percentage. For those needing healing, close the eyes and speak softly, internally:

"I see all the people standing in front of me. There is a strong white light of healing covering their entire bodies. This healing light penetrates each cell in their bodies, healing all cells from head to toe."

Fix the intention and concentrate on the white light, representing the power of healing.

MORE INSIGHT INTO HEALING

"The invisible forces are ever working for man who is always 'pulling the strings' himself, though he does not know it. Owing to the vibratory power of words, whatever man voices, he begins to attract."

The Game of Life, FLORENCE SCOVEL SHINN

Our world has changed drastically. We no longer have to hunt wild animals for our food, in a scenario where the predator would sometimes turn around and hunt the human instead, where the prey and the victim were interchangeable, depending on who got the upper hand.

Today's predators we can no longer escape from. Lawyers, accountants, bankers and bureaucrats can target us through phone calls, emails and mail-outs. Issues can no longer be dealt with in a discreet time period, they are present all the time. These are big changes and ones which we are still learning to cope with. The very problems which cause us the most stress are the ones that are outside our control. Faceless companies supply our homes and offices with power for heating and lighting, so in times of crises when power goes off, we have no control. Machines that used to help us now have us working for them.

The rules of modern life are changing so fast, that what a graduate learnt at university may be out of date by the time they start their career. We can now foresee problems that don't even exist at the present moment. This is when our body's power can be misapplied; our brain sees a social problem as a physical threat. We are manipulated by political, religious and commercial leaders and we in turn manipulate others. When this manipulation makes us feel guilty, frustrated or incomplete, it causes stress, and results in inappropriate actions. The human body and mind have not had time to adapt to these new levels of threat, not had time to learn to differentiate between physical and mental responses, or the fact that making decisions can sometimes turn out to be harmful.

Many diseases today are produced by people overreacting. Heart disease, ulcers, high blood pressure and many others are powerful physiological responses which have been activated by psychological threats. If our body's defence system is overreacting, we need to change our exposure to stress and our mental response to it. The allopathic method of treating symptom instead of cause offers only temporary solutions. The very best thing we can do for ourselves is to understand your own weak points. Everybody has them, and once we are aware of them, we can guard and maintain our own health easier.

Here are some of the emotions or situations that can lead to certain weaknesses or diseases:

Asthma: a domineering mother, a weak father. Not releasing anger, fears, tears and joy. A lonely, oversensitive soul who doesn't express emotions.

Ulcers: dependent on the mother, needs lots of love. Ambitious and hardworking.

Depressive: Feel helpless, inadequate, ineffectual, think little of themselves, introvert, no sense of humour, hard to adapt to change. Likely to become ill in a crisis. Rigid inhibition of self-expression.

Heart Attack: those who are aggressive, impatient, competitive, anxious to succeed. Forever competing with the father. No matter how successful they are, it rarely fulfils their ambition (it's not how successful you are, but how successful you think you are).

Eczema: Sensitive people similar to asthma people, repress their emotions, keep their anger to themselves and bottle up emotions.

Arthritis: Tend to be timid, shy, and dissatisfied with their own work. Bad taskmasters. Come from unhappy homes, where one parent may be hard, domineering and cruel. Inferiority complex, likes to conform, and feels helpless. Difficulty in expressing self.

Colitis: Shy, dependent, passive and anxious. Indecision, immaturity, avoiding conflict.

Cancer: It is known today that people who are prone to cancer try too hard to please the world. When they fail, as they surely will, cancer can be the result. Unhappy childhoods, lack of love, loneliness. They tend to give more than they take and unselfishly please others.

Migraine: Driven by guilt and the need to satisfy their own over-demanding conscience. Perfectionists, ambitious and anxious to please, neat and orderly. Rage when things go wrong leads to migraine.

Hay Fever: Timid nervous people, lack confidence, and can be obsessive. Badly affected by crises, trauma. Symptoms tend to worsen when things are bad.

Neck: Pain in front of the neck stands for something or someone that is ahead of you. Pain in the back of neck shows there are problems with you, or someone, or something in the past. Leave the past and let your future unfold. Learn to trust in what is ahead.

A woman will feel illness on the left side of her head, where negative thoughts about the self reside. The right side of the head is where negative thoughts about others are held.

When a man feels pain on his right side, they indicate negative thoughts about the self. The left side of the head is where thoughts about others lie. A headache is the first sign of negative thoughts. Pain in the back of the head is from negative thoughts from the past.

Heart Disease: blocking out intimacy or love from their lives.

Lower Back Pain: persistent financial worries.

Blood Disorder: not enough joy or ideas circulating in the body.

This list is not complete but gives an idea of where to take action. Remember that even small aches and pains in our body should not be ignored. Your body is telling you something. Know your weak points and pay attention to symptoms: headache; skin rash; indigestion; wheezing; diarrhoea; chest pains; palpitations; insomnia; irritability. All of these show the beginnings of physical damage, indicating that you have reached your stress limit. In such cases, you need to pay attention and apply simple first-aid techniques: tense and release the muscles in your body, from your toes to the top of your head. Relax your mind and remember that you have an imagination powerful enough to control your physical destiny. Everyone has. Appreciate the power of positive emotion.

When to see your doctor?

» If you have unexplained pain for 5 or more days.

» Bleeding anywhere

» Loss or gain of weight, lumps or swelling

» Warts or skin blemishes, changing size or colour, or bleeding

» New symptoms from pre-treated areas

» Mental conditions, confusion, paranoia, depression

We can be sure that negative thoughts cause pain and illness while positive thoughts bring healing to body, mind, soul. While accepting that illness is part of life on earth and our journey through it, we can also begin to understand that health is in our heads not in our bodies. Since we have accepted the polarities of health and illness, we can begin to take blame away from ourselves, since it will only exacerbate our discomfort. Treat yourself as you would treat a friend. It's your thoughts that create your life. Remember that negative thoughts create distress, depression, conflict, crisis, failure, pain, illness, injuries. The more serious the illness the more assistance you will need from other sources, so you really want to pay attention to your symptoms and your thoughts and catch things in time.

Remember that you are in control of your body. Tell it what you want and make sure it does it. Focus on health, not the problem. What you think is what you get. If what you say is different to what you think, it is the thought that rules, so think positively. If you are stressed, this is best dealt with by relaxing. Start by deep breathing and pour the oxygen into yourself. Breathe in positive, breathe out negative energy and try meditation.

Visualisation is a method used by high performance sports people to accomplish the greatest feats of physical endurance. The body doesn't know the difference between what is imaginary and what is real. Picture in your mind what you want. Use visualisation for healing, believing that your body becomes whatever you tell it to be. Ask your body to release all problems to the earth. Remove all dark energies from your aura and send back clear white light.

Releasing is another method we can use to help us rid ourselves of clogged energies. These can also be dealt with using the clearing techniques of dowsing, by asking that they be removed from the body, mind, and soul. Remember that it is possible to release what is causing the problem. Get rid of karmic energy by asking in God's name: "In God's name I ask that _____ (symptom/illness) leave me now." Do not focus on the problem or else it will not leave you, but only make you worse.

Locating Pain: Find the pain with your finger, males use the first finger (negative polarity) females with their second finger (negative polarity). Place the negative finger on the place of pain and say "I demand that this pain leave my body now." Then males change to second finger (positive polarity) and females to the first finger (positive polarity) and say "Please replace this energy with energy of the highest appropriate level, for the good of all." Repeat this process 3 or 4 times. Once you learn to use a pendulum, this job will be so much easier.

Guidance

Listen to your body. The longer negative energy remains in your body, the longer you ignore it, the more intense it gets. The sooner you recognise the pain, the easier it is to heal and to start thinking positively again. Think through the pain with positive thoughts. Negative thoughts lower your energy. When you discover what is causing your problems you change your life or change your thoughts. If you don't pay attention to how you feel your body will tell you when you aren't doing it right. Know that you can heal yourself.

"I release all past and present _____" (e.g. pain, illness, sickness etc.)

When Others Get Sick

Always think positive thoughts when you are with someone who is sick. Do not accept responsibility for the outcome, you are only a facilitator sending the energy from the higher self to the recipient.

"Let go and let God do the work".

Good health is for everybody. The first law of medicine: Remove the Cause. The real disease is not the outward physical but the inner mental state. The cause of most sickness is in the mind, and can be found in the emotions: fear, jealousies, anxieties, frustration, traumatic experiences from the past. Even the advertising we see around modern medicine is fear based, so you must be vigilant as to how your emotions can be manipulated so that you know what is happening, and counteract it. "Remove the Cause" means that we must learn to erase the destructive thought pattern before we can hope to eradicate the physical symptoms.

Awakening

We all walk around in an unconscious state of mind, almost as if we were asleep. The first step in awakening is a process of observation. Non-judgementally just being aware of what is going on. Notice what makes you happy, sad, angry, bored, excited. When you sleep, activate the sleep portion of your mind (the subconscious) and allow it to release the enormous store of information/power that it holds, the power of the psychic realm.

These steps will help you achieve increased satisfaction in life and psychic growth. It all begins, must begin, with self-knowledge. Self-healing begins with self-observation.

Pain and Disease

Pain and disease are the result of a disruption or imbalance. It may be a single upset, a series of small irritations, or same old forgotten conflict that was never resolved. Or just some tiresome person who annoys you. These disturbances will show up in our psychic or astral body, before reaching our physical body, allowing you to diagnose illness before it happens.

The process of being ill is part of the process of being well. Sometimes you may have to go through with the illness. To recover, one must ask: "What does this body need to regain its psychic balance?"

If a person has a sore back, they should have a conversation with their back: "Okay back, what is going on? What do you want from me that you are not getting?" The answer will be: "Love me" and your reply: "I love you, you're my one and only back." The response may well be: "You don't love me the right way – you walk funny, you sit funny, you never give me a rest, always doing, doing, doing."

Every part of your body needs to change position and unwind from time to time, you must remember to recharge yourself.

Deep Relaxation: The Healing State

What we are aiming to do here is to enable you to meditate and enter a state of deep relaxation without going to sleep. We want you to reduce your brain wave vibrations down from the 14 to 21 vibrations per second (Hertz) of a normal waking state, to the 7 to 14 Hz in what is called the Alpha state. Alpha is the best state to attain in order to be able to programme yourself to health and happiness. This is when good things happen to the body. The body is reactivated, blood pressure normalizes, and the client may gain control of parts of their body they were having problems with.

Learn to use your mind to resolve any health problems. It's the mind that heals.

Before we start doing any healing, we must be completely relaxed:

» Sit in a comfortable chair. Close your eyes and look up through your forehead.

» Count slowly back from one hundred down to one.

» Relax and bring peaceful thoughts into your mind.

» Think and repeat: "Every day in every way, I'm getting better and better."

» When you get to the number five, start thinking about opening your eyes.

» When you are at one, say "I am wide awake and life is great."

Do this every day first thing in the morning, then another two times throughout the day.

That we want to achieve is to have this routine – and these positive affirmations – imprinted on your mind. The more you repeat the procedure, it will become easier for you to remember.

» Do the count down from 100 for 12 days

» Then reduce the numbers so you count down from 50 for 12 days

» Then from 25 for twelve days

After those thirty-six days of training, you will only need to count down from 10 to reach an Alpha state.

After Reaching Alpha

The best healing is done when the healer is in the Alpha state, and the person being healed is in a relaxed and receptive state for the healing to work. Healing relies on all people involved taking their bodies to a relaxed state, thereby making it easier for the healing energy to repair the body. We start the healing by doing the countdown exercises as outlined earlier, and having worked our way through relaxing each area of the body starting from the head to the toes.

Near the end of the exercise, you then concentrate on the part of your body that needs healing, move your hands to the area and send the energy through the place that needs attention, saying: "Remove this pain and problem from my mind, my body, my soul."

You must always think of yourself as already healed while doing this. It's all in the mind.

How To Do a Simple Healing

» Sit in a straight-backed chair, feet on the ground. Arms and legs uncrossed, hands on thighs, palms up.
» Close your eyes, relax, clear your mind, with your full attention on yourself.
» Ground yourself.
» Start at your head and follow your aura down your body.
» If you visualise cool/dark/sticky energy then visualise orange light flowing through the area and cleaning out that energy.
» When the body is cleared of this energy, send clean golden light to cover it completely.
» Open your eyes, clasp your hands, sit quietly, bend over and let your head hang between your knees.

Running Energy Through Your Body

» Sit in a straight-backed chair, close your eyes, relax, clear your mind, ground yourself.
» Maintain grounded focus on feet chakras (arch of feet).
» Imagine the light brown energy of planet earth drawing up through your legs, thighs, and into your first chakra (root).
» Imagine this energy passing up through your body to the seventh chakra (crown).
» Then passing into the aura and hands.
» Now bring this energy back down through the body.
» Imagine golden light flowing through the crown chakra and down your body to the solar plexus chakra.
» Let the energy mix with the energy that you bring up through your body to the solar plexus from the ground.
» Keep circulating it and then send it into the ground.

Opening/Closing Chakras

» Sit in psychic posture, with a clear mind, and grounded.
» Focus on first chakra (root) and imagine it opening up like an iris, as wide as it can go.
» Now imagine it slowly closing till it is completely shut.
» Imagine this happening three times.
» Do this imagining exercise to all the chakras. (Eventually you will be able to do this at will.)
» Take a last look at your chakras and decide how open you wish them to be: 10 per cent, 20 per cent, whatever is needed to let the energy flow.
» Now come out of trance.

Honing Your Psychic Ability

» Sit in psychic position, feet on ground, legs and arms uncrossed, palms facing upwards. Stay grounded.

» Open your eyes and look at all four corners of the ceiling.

» Pick one corner and close your eyes again.

» Imagine that you are in that corner looking down at your body in the chair for a few moments.

» Imagine your aura and what it looks like.

» Imagine you are back in your body, inside your head. How does it feel being back in your body?

» Go back and forth between the corner and your body several times.

» Come out of trance.

Colour Meditation

» Run a selected coloured energy up from the ground through your feet and legs, and bring the same colour down through your chakras.

» Use the chakra colours Red, Orange, Yellow, Green, Blue, Indigo, Violet, choosing one colour at a time and taking turns at circulating them through your whole body one at a time for 30 seconds to 1 minute each.

» Come out of the trance.

» Always clasp hands when finished, to stop energy flowing out randomly.

» Bending over with your head between your legs allows excess psychic energy to leave your body.

Psychic Cords

Remember that you can't receive another person's psychic cords unless you are willing to do so. No one can do anything to you psychically. It always takes two.

- If the psychic cord attaches to the First Chakra (Root) it undermines your survival. Such a cord is only permissible if the person attaching is sick or a baby. If friends or lovers attach this cord to you, you need to get rid of it.

- Second Chakra (Sacral) – I am interested in you. Give me your emotion, pay attention to my emotion.
  Energy could be draining from you. Cut the cord to stop it.

- Third Chakra (Solar Plexus) – Energy centre. I want some of your energy, my own is not enough or I would rather operate on yours than use my own.
  Remove cord, cut it. A strong cord of this type would create a tight sensation in your stomach.

- Fourth Chakra (Heart) – Love and affinity. I love you, I like you. Please yourself if you remove them or let them stay.

- Fifth Chakra (Throat) – Communication. I want to communicate with you. I want to talk to you. Or I want to stop you talking.v
  A large cord can cause you to have an ache in your throat.

- Sixth Chakra (Third Eye) – Clairvoyant. I'm in your head, thinking of you, wondering what you are thinking of. Causes a headache.

- Seventh Chakra (Crown) – Knowingness/Intuition. I want to control you. I want you to follow my teachings.

- Hand Chakras – Do it my way, do it for me. It affects creativity.

- Feet Chakras – Dislocates your grounding and makes you vague and spaced out.

How to Pull Cords from Yourself

» Sit in the psychic posture, close your eyes, clear your mind and become grounded.

» Follow the 'How to do a Simple Healing' process.

» Follow the 'Open and Close Chakras' process.

» Free Chakras of cords by making the cutting action with open hands and chopping the cords that might be attached.

» Visualise clear clean neutral golden energy around and through you.

» Start at the head and work towards the feet.

» Next, smooth out your aura.

» Come out of trance, wash your face and hands, have a cup of tea.

» Be nice to yourself for the rest of the day.

Healing Auras

» Ground yourself.

» Paint a black silhouette of a person.

» Observe a large thin halo around them.

» Allow the white halo to become coloured.

» Dissolve and repeat on another friend.

» Come out of Alpha state.

Severe Psychic Disorders

» Send them to a qualified psychotherapist.

» You can help by doing basic healing and distant healing.

» Some people are attached to their illness, they have a 'hidden agenda'.

» You cannot heal a person who doesn't want to be healed.

» Psychic healing is about helping someone to heal themselves. Ask: "Do they want to be healed?"

Healing from Drugs

» Ground the person well, through their first chakra and through their feet.

» Clean out their first chakra and fill the void with gold and blue energy.

» Have them do something that makes their body feel real without drugs (sport, creativity etc).

After Suffering a 'Psychic Whack'

Say you are crossing the road and a passing driver abuses you for no reason. Or the same scenario occurs in a supermarket. This is called a 'psychic whack' and can send you out of your body and put you in your head space. You lose track of where you are. The solution is to run some healing energy through yourself, pulling off any cords and grounding yourself.

WHEN YOU GET STUCK IN A READING:

» Reground yourself and the other person.

» Raise your energy levels above the person being healed.

» Dissolve all the pictures you have made.

» Close down your sacral chakra.

» Start again.

What to Remember in Faith Healing:

- Faith is belief which is not based on proof.
- Belief is a conviction of the truth or reality without knowledge.
- If you think you can earn $15,000, that is all you will be able to earn.
- If you think you can earn $75,000 that's what you'll earn.
- If you believe eating dog food will make you healthy, eat it.
- If your ideas clash with The Word, suffer the guilt.
- Isolate yourself from your the person being healed, so they don't own you.
- The less the healer cares about the results of his healing, the more potent a healer he will be.
- The most powerful healings are affected from a state of pure love.
- Work from the fourth chakra (heart) or the throat (or both), loving for love's sake alone.
- If the healer's energies go to supporting his ego, his mind is elsewhere. Put aside personal desire.
- You only need the intent that the healing will take place.

You don't have to cut cords or make up roses, psychic space or colours. All you have to do to effect healing is to forget the details of the person's disease; just intend that they be well. If your friend doesn't feel well, let him feel unwell. Since he doesn't feel well already, letting him feel that way should be easy. But letting things be isn't easy. Letting things be the way they are is extremely hard because everyone has a picture of how things should be, or how things will be when they are well. You must avoid resistance because you become what you resist, and other people, the world and the cosmos also become what you resist. When you do not resist the way things are, those things have the psychic space to finish being the way they are, and to move on to being whatever they are next. To affect a healing you have to surrender.

Remembering to Stay Positive

It cannot be repeated enough that health is our natural state of being. It is down to us to make the positive choice and to reject the presence of sickness and the negative thoughts that keep us bound to ill-health. The very best thing we can achieve in life is to maintain a healthy mind and body, enabling us to progress spiritually, and to die a natural death when our time comes.

Every one of us can remain healthy, happy, relieved of stress, anger, greed and fear. Every one of us can understand health and prevent disease by following some simple methods. The methods we are advocating are not complex or difficult to understand, but only ask for a little time and commitment on your part in order to enforce new habits of health that can benefit you and those around you. We have been led to believe that material comforts and money will fulfil our desires but such promises are slowly losing their validity as humanity lurches towards societal and environmental disaster brought on by pure materialism. Now is the time when we are all being called upon to look after our health, in the understanding that material satisfaction will follow.

What we are advocating is not any kind of religion. We are simply pointing out what all peoples have known since the beginning of time, but which our present materialist mindset has tried to make us forget: there is a cosmic energy that is beyond us, greater than us, and prepared to help us. The only way to make use of this free, benign energy is to ask for its help. Ask and you will receive. However, we must make sure that we receive the energy in the proper and beneficial way, knowing that faith must be our most loyal ally. From the highest ranking official to the simplest and humblest human being, faith is the vehicle that will allow us to let healing into our lives.

We suggest that you try this simple, tried and tested programme, but first please take heed of these five points of preparation:

1. Always think through the issue. Hold the belief that the person to be healed, whether that be another or yourself, is already healed. We must maintain a positive mind.

2. Understand that healing always involves the body, mind and soul. Contrary to what you have been taught or told, illness is not always in the body. The healer's job is to find out where the illness is and help the other person (remember that it is the other person that does the healing, we healers are merely channelers).

3. Please, please, please, release all negative emotions. They are the main reason that healings don't take place. Positive emotions are what both the healer and the other person need.

4. For best healing results the patient must bring their energy into the energy of the healer. They must both be bathed in positive

energy. Again, we have to repeat that it is not the healer's energy that does the healing, the healer's job is to channel the greater energy through to the other person. Healers never use their own energy, as this would simply run them down and they would forever be trying to recuperate.

5. Understand that your mind controls your body. Send your body healthy thoughts and in time it will respond and you will see the results. Don't be trapped in a negative pattern, change your thought pattern to positive, or else you will remain a negative thinker always in need of medicines and hospitals.

PERSONAL EXPERIENCES AND TECHNIQUE

Distant Healing

Now is the time to tell a couple of stories about some of my experiences. The first story I'd like to recount concerns Johnnie, who was having problems with flies in his house and asked if I could do something about them. Johnnie lived 60 odd kilometres away from me, but I agreed to clear them, in what is called distant healing. What I needed was a photo of a fly or flies to use as a witness in order to move them on. They were emailed to me and when I took the first photo off the printer, I was dismayed to see that the first picture was of a dead fly. Of course, there would be no need to remove dead flies from his house, so I was pleased to see that the second photo was of a live fly, which meant I could now start using my magic. With the photo in front of me, I started a conversation with the flies. I thanked them for the job they had done and suggested that now would be a good time to move on to better pastures. Notice how even with a fly, for all its faults, I never at any time became aggressive.

In a short time, Johnnie called to tell me that the flies had gone, and I was chuffed to hear that the clearing worked. However, talking to Johnnie later, he told me the flies did leave the house, but when he entered the outhouse the following morning, he found about a dozen of the same flies inside! In actual fact, the healing had worked, the flies got the message and left the house, but we had forgotten about the outhouse. What we should have done in this case was to clear both buildings, remembering to specify " I clear all buildings".

I should make a note here that working with a photo makes the process easier. A lot of dowsers use photos if they cannot be present at the scene of the healing, and it can also work with a person. Just make sure that when using a photo that it is only of the person you are healing. Do not try to cut a person's photo off a group photo because the energies of the group are still with the person.

In another interesting situation, Peter rang me and asked me to clear negative energies from his flat. He lives about 12 kilometres from my home and while talking to him on the phone I checked his unit for geopathic stress (negative ley lines going through his property). I did this by taking a piece of A4 paper, imaging it is the unit where he lives, then using my left hand and with the pendulum in my right hand, I let my hand wander around the paper looking for negative energies or geopathic stress. Through this method I discovered that there were a few issues which could be causing problems. Now Peter told me he is in a large complex with about 18 units, where members of a bike gang and drug dealers lived, so I offered to clear the whole block and see what happened.

Everything in this world has a vibrational level, plants, animals, humans, rocks, steel, etc. These vibrations are critical to the universe and to ourselves. Ancients were very particular where they built their houses, and understood where the bad energy in the land was located, and looked for the sites of beneficial energies. They knew where and how to find geopathic disturbances in the form of underground streams, unhealthy mineral concentrations, fault lines, quarries and mine workings. Geopathic stress can be a drain on your energies, impeding your immune system as it battles with the geopathic stress instead of doing the repair work on your body that it's meant to. Sleeping in an area of geopathic energy is particularly detrimental to health. Over time this allows illness to creep in.

If you are sleeping in an area like this and not getting enough rest, you may notice that when sleeping away from home you sleep very soundly, and should take this as an indication you need to check your house.

Peter rang me back some days later and told me he didn't feel any difference in the energy levels of the unit. Now remember I cleared the total complex. While talking to him, I decided to check my work over throughout the complex again, getting the answers from the pendulum that I had indeed been successful. Now when working in clearing a home, the first place I check is the person's bed, because this is where they spend most of their time. I checked his bed again and found that there was still geopathic stress going through it. I couldn't work out what had happened, the complex was clear but his unit was not cleared. I decided to clear his unit on its own this time and see what happened. He then gave me his address and while explaining the layout to me, he said there were 3 large complexes on the property. This lit a lightbulb in my mind: I had obviously cleared one of the large units, but not the one he was living in! I am sure when he rings next week, he will have noticed the difference.

Both these stories illustrate that if something is not working right, you need to ask more questions, because the answer is there somewhere. They also show the power of energy healing – you just believe it and it will happen.

My Healing Procedure

Germs do not harm us if we are well. Viruses and bacteria do no harm to us as long as we are well, because we have our defence system to protect us. Imagine that we are just like meat and fruit: if we are not protected, we start to go bad and decay. This happens quickly with meat but takes longer with fruit. Fruit decay starts in one small place and slowly expands to cover the entire fruit. Often humans are more like fruit, in that illness happens slowly. It's not because we have the flu that we are sick. It's because we are sick that we have the flu, we are not fully alive with all our vitality. The first place to look when illness strikes is your toxicity levels.

All disease comes from three places: poor diet and lack of exercise or unhappiness of the mind and spirit. It is often this unhappiness (in the form of unresolved trauma) that can be the hardest to tackle, but again faith is all important here. We must believe in healing and know that it is going to happen. God loves you and can heal you. For those who are not comfortable with using God, I will use the word Life, so it will be God/Life.

I feel that nobody should discount the information because they have had a bad experience in relationship with the concept of God/Life. I like to use the phrase 'God of Light', as to me this signifies a positive outside energy far greater than us, that is there to be used by us all.

Healing the Client

The first question to ask the pendulum is, "Does this person want to be healed?" If I get the 'yes' answer, I carry on. If the pendulum indicates a 'no', we still have options. We can then ask the pendulum "Are there any energy blocks in the body, mind, soul of this client?" If so, we clear it. If not, ask "Are there any negative energies, entities, non-beneficial spirits attached to their body, mind, soul?" If so, clear them and then ask again: "Does this Person want to be healed?" If 'yes', carry on. However, in the case of another 'no', be aware that you can also ask the Higher Self through the pendulum: "Higher Self, can this person be healed?" If the answer is 'yes', you have the okay to continue.

Remember, if the client is not inclined towards healing the healing is not going to happen.

If you keep getting a 'no', do not proceed.

Next, we assess the client's energy vibration level. This is a pre-set figure that the dowser sets with his pendulum, which is programmed and therefore stays with the pendulum (see chapter 'The What and How of Dowsing'). Say the client's energy vibration levels are low, then the dowser must remove any blockages otherwise the healing will not happen.

1. "Please remove all energy blockages from _____'s body, mind, soul." The pendulum rotates anticlockwise till it stops.

2. Now the dowser raises the energy vibration levels. "Raise the energy vibration levels to the highest possible level, for the good of all." The Pendulum rotates clockwise until it stops.

Repeat both steps one and two till the pendulum no longer rotates in the anticlockwise direction. Then you know that the negative energy has been removed. At the end of this procedure, check the energy vibration levels to make sure that they are equal to, or higher than, the pre-set figure mentioned before. Say 'Thank you'.

Now we check the Life Force of the client. Here we are checking if there are any earlier life issues that need to be dealt with. Basically, we are going to go back in time to when the issue happened, then back a wee bit further to bring this energy forward to the present day. This helps to release the past issue that needs to be cleared. With some people you may have to go back to a past life to find the issue.

It's a good idea at this point to check whether there are any negative energies, entities or non-beneficial spirits attached to them. Ask your outer energy source if they have the ability to remove them. If you get a 'no', please beware, you may need professional help to remove them (see chapter 'Dowsing and Radionics').

We have now handled the big stuff.

Now for a healing where we are sending healing to clients who have an illness. Hold the pendulum in your hand and scan the diagram of the body we have prepared on page 179 with the other hand, looking for swings of the pendulum that indicate negative areas in the body. When you find any, hold your free hand over the area and watch the pendulum rotate anticlockwise (removing bad energy) till it stops, then the pendulum will rotate clockwise till it naturally stops (sending healing).

When someone contacts me for healing, this is how I would normally proceed:

Summary

1. Check their home and any land around it for geopathic stress, negative energies, entities and non-beneficial spirits.

2. Do the same for their place of work.

3. Do any clearing work that needs to be done in these places.

4. Ask, "Does this person want to be healed?"
    If the answer is 'no', I then check to see if there are any negative energies, entities, or non-beneficial spirits that need to be cleared before I get the go-ahead to do the healing work. At this point, I dowse, saying "Please remove all blockages from _____'s body, mind, soul."

    NOTE: Do not proceed with any healing until you get a 'yes' response to the first question. Some people, for their own reasons, do not want to be healed. The choice is theirs.

5. Healing work includes working directly with the person present or distant healing, which can be done anywhere in the world. This can be hands on, hands above the body, pendulum, or radionics.

6. Balance the chakras, check the energy vibration levels, life force, and aura. Check the meridians and organs that need clearing.

7. While you are working with the patient you might make time to heal any pets living with them.

8. Test their food, "Is this food good for _____."

9. Check the energy of their friendship and/or working group.

People ask me what made me take up dowsing, and I always reply that I don't really know how I started. I do remember that at the beginning, I played around with a pendulum and just persisted with it for four months before I was able to get a yes/no response. After that, I bought and read dowsing books that got me interested in trying my hand at locating different energies, mainly in the ground.

While practising with my pendulum I would ask it questions that I knew were correct, like "Is my name David?" and it would give me a 'yes'. Then I would ask "Is my name Ralph?" and it would give me a 'yes', which is also true because my name is Ralph David.

Following on from this, I might ask the test question, " Is my name Jenny?" and get a 'no'. This is also right. While you are practising with the pendulum even if you know that the question is wrong, still ask it and see what answer you get. Every good dowser will tell you that the more you practise the better you'll become at it. Please, please, practise, practise, practise.

Next, I learnt to use the divining rods, looking for drains, water mains, phone lines, power lines, underground streams and anything that may be located underground This led me to studying ley lines in the ground and how to remove the bad energy (see below).

At this stage, I signed up for a Raymon Grace's Dowsing Weekend over the internet and I thank him for making dowsing look so simple and easy. It taught me that there is nothing you can't dowse for, as long as you are only asking for a yes/no answer, percentage of, or number between, say, 1 and 50.

So much for how I got here. If you were contacting me regarding a problem you may have at home or work, this is how I would approach your situation:

While we were discussing the situation – be that over the phone or at your home – I would be checking with the pendulum as we were talking, trying to identify what issues need attention. It is important to state that I have 'no skin in the game'; that I am totally independent and not affected by what has been going on with this situation, so may be able to find something that the client has not thought about.

This is the best advice for all people who want to be able to dowse. Do not at any time think or wish the answer – you are using intuition so let it give you the answer. Do not use the frontal lobe of your brain, get in a relaxed state and let the answers come to you.

While doing this important work make sure that you relax, take two deep breaths occasionally, turn your brain off and only think of what you are doing. Follow this same procedure for a place of work, commercial building, etc. The interesting thing here is that a business may be having problems in one area of the factory, and it can show up as having plenty of geopathic stress lines which are draining the people that work in this area. You can also dowse the geopathic stress lines in an outside area like a park or a garden and remove them from the land.

• • •

To end this book, is to state that this is not the end. The art of dowsing and radiesthesia are an on-going process of learning through study and practise.

Please find me at my website *www.selfhealingcentre.com* to access more information, download more rosettes with healing for specific conditions, and to join online courses and training.

References

Bailes, Fredrick. *Your Mind Can Heal You* (Published 2004 by Kessinger Publishing, 1971)

Bailey, Arthur. *Anyone Can Dowse for Better Health* (1998, Foulsham)

Baltasar-Schwartz, Francis. *Attitude is Everything* http://blasiegroup.sas.upenn.edu/strzalka/attitude.html

Branan, Barbara Ann – www.jmshah.com

Coldwell, Dr Leonard. *The Only Answer to Cancer: Defeating the Root Cause of all Disease* (21st Century Press, 2009)

Coleman, Dr Vernon. *Body Power: Secret of Self-Healing* (Gardners Books; 1994)

Compassionate Frome Project, UK

Dethlefsen, Thorwald. *Healing Power of Illness: Understanding what your Symptoms are Telling You* (Sentient Publications; 2016)

Francis, Raymond. *The Great American Health Hoax: The Surprising Truth about how Modern Medicine keeps you Sick* (Health Communications Inc 2015)

Gerber, Richard. *Vibrational Medicine: The #1 Handbook of Subtle-Energy Therapies* (Bear & Company, 2001)

Grace, Raymon. https://www.raymongrace.us/about-dowsing.html

Hay, Louise. *You Can Heal Your Life* (Hay House Inc. January 1, 1984)

Hills, Christopher. Various, including *Supersenonics—The Science of Radiational Paraphysics* (1975)

Hollingshead, Sheila. *The Pendulum: Making Energy Visible* https://b-ok.global/ireader/5362046

Holzer, Hans. *Beyond Medicine: The Facts about Unorthodox and Psychic Healing* (Ballantine Books, 1974)

Johnson, Spencer. *The Present: The Gift That Makes You Happier and More Successful at Work and in Life,* Today! (Crown Business, 2003)

Imber, Gerald. *Genius on the Edge: The Bizarre Double Life of Dr. William Stewart Halsted* (Kaplan Publishing, 2011)

Kermani, Dr Kai. *Distant Healing* – https://www.healingwithdrkermani.co.uk

Knowles, Dan. *Road Map to Ultimate Health* – available from Beyond Health – https://beyondhealth.com/health-roadmaps/

Moloch, Brother. *The Radionics Primer* https://www.rad111.com

Moretto, Ruggero. *Basic Course of Radionics and Radiesthesia* http://www.biolifestyle.org/dowsing.pdf

Mister, Teri. http://transformationaltruth.com

Myss, Carolyn. *Why People Don't Heal and How they Can* (Harmony; First Paperback Edition (September 23, 1998)

Patten, Leslie. *Biocircuits: Amazing New Tools for Energy Health* (H J Kramer; 1st U.S. Edition, 1988)

Ramacharaka, Yogi. *The Science of Psychic Healing* (Yoga Publication Society, 1987)

Rife, Royal Raymond. *The Rife Handbook of Frequency Therapy and Holistic Health: an integrated approach for cancer and other diseases* – 5th Edition in PDF format available from https://www.researchgate.net

Rothkranz, Markus. *Bacteria, Virus and Cancer are not the Bad Guys* (article) https://www.markusrothkranz.com

Sampson, Brenda. *New Zealand's Greatest Doctor Ulrich Williams of Wanganui: a Surgeon who became a Naturopath* (Zealand Publishing House, 2003)

Silva, Jose / Stone, Robert. *You the Healer: The World-Famous Silva Method on How to Heal Yourself and Others* (HJ Kramer, 1992)

Woods, Walt. *Letter to Robin: a Mini Course in Pendulum Dowsing,* available from https://lettertorobin.files.wordpress.com/2016/06/rbn_10_4_english.pdf

Sai Sanjeevini Healing https://www.saisanjeevini.org

DIAGRAMS

1. *Body diagram front (clean)*

2. *Body diagram back (clean)*

3. *Body diagram – front with meridians*

4. *Body diagram – back with meridians*

5. *Dowsing chart*

6. *Radionics Rosette (clean)*

Working with the Radionics Rosette:
If someone is not feeling well or they have an illness, it follows that their energy then vibrates at a lower level. To help with the healing we must do our best to raise the person's energy levels. The energy that is stored in this rosette is sufficient to do this work for you. One must constantly keep in mind that the person sending the healing is not doing the healing: the healing comes from a higher source and through the rosette. It is the universal energy of life, of the universe. It took me a while to believe this, but trust me it works and we are giving you the opportunity to try it for yourself for free.

This rosette is an elaborated magnetron design for amplifying energies, based on the work of Christopher Hills and drawing on the power of the Great Pyramid.

Rosettes with healing for specific conditions

These are a set of different healing scenarios. Find one that you think may help yourself or others you are concerned for. Print it off and then write the person's name on a piece of paper and place the paper in the centre of the rosette. Leave for at least one minute and then let the energy do the rest. This can be repeated several times and is the best way to send a healing. Don't worry if you leave the name on the rosette, although the healing won't be quite as effective as taking it on and off. Always say to yourself, "This healing is being done for The Good of All"

7. *Healing Combination No. 4 – Back problems*

8. *Healing Combination No. 10 – To increase brain power*

9. *Healing Combination No. 12 – Kidney Cleanse*

10. *Healing Combination No. 15 – Diabetes*

11. *Healing Combination No. 24 – Headaches*

12. *Healing Combination No. 25 – Heart issues*

13. *Healing Combination No. 27 – Liver complaints*

14. *Healing Combination No. 31 – Infection and inflammation/fever*

15. *Healing Combination No. 40 – Addictions*

16. *Healing Combination No. 59 – Removal of negative emotions*

17. *Healing Combination No. 70 – Total System Tonic (with clearing of toxins)*

NB: Each of these graphs contains the cure for blockages, toxins, deficiency, psychological, physical, genetic and medical causes.

1. *Body diagram front (clean)*   2. *Body diagram back (clean)*

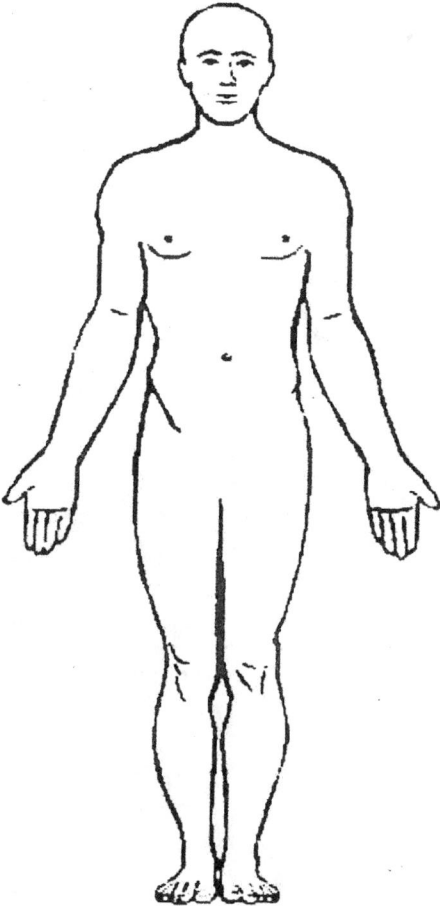

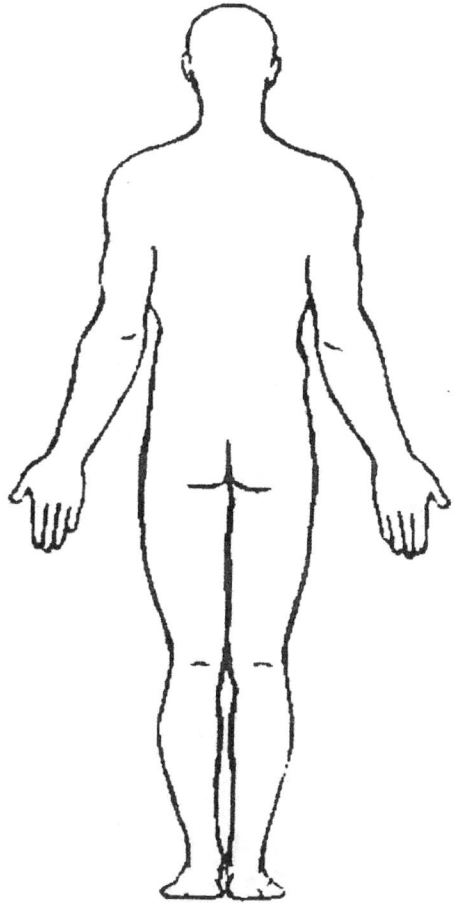

3. *Body diagram
front with meridians*

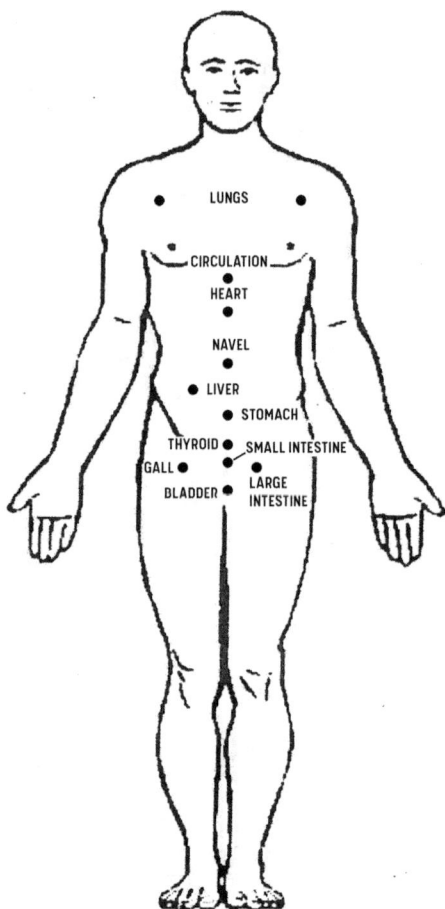

4. *Body diagram
back with meridians*

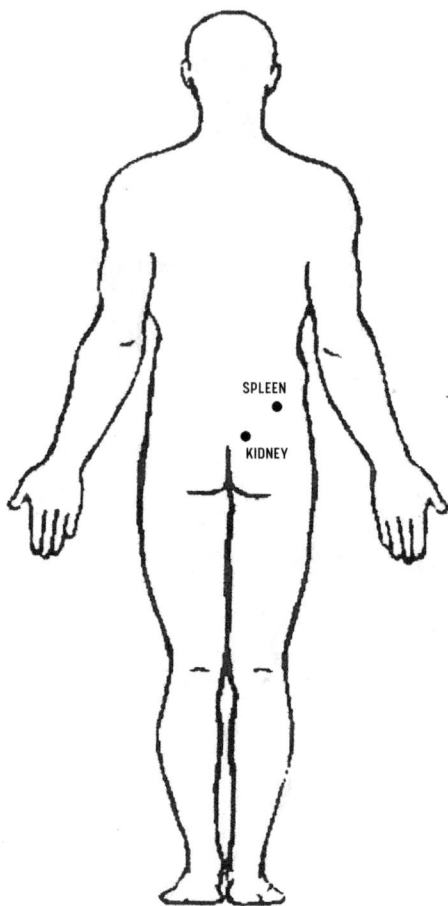

3. Front labels:

LUNGS

CIRCULATION

HEART

NAVEL

LIVER

STOMACH

THYROID

SMALL INTESTINE

GALL

BLADDER

LARGE
INTESTINE

4. Back labels:

SPLEEN

KIDNEY

5. Dowsing chart

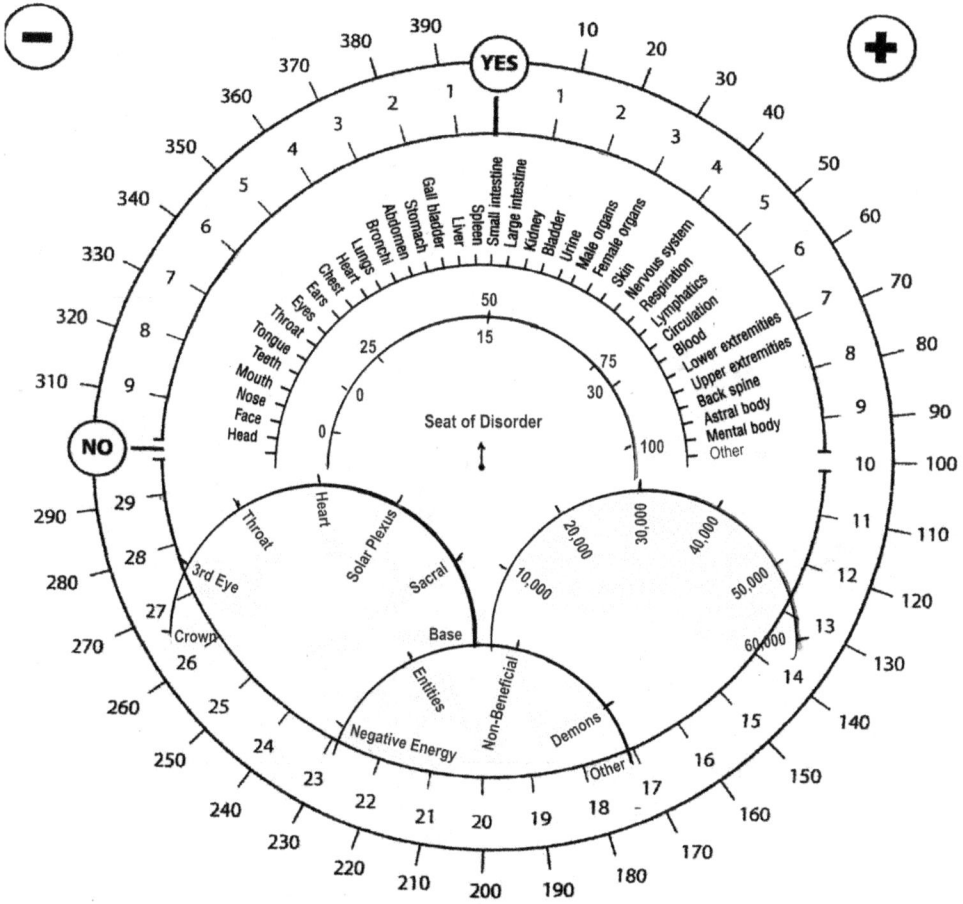

Created by Walt Woods and adapted by Raymon Grace. Used by dowsers all over the world. For more information about dowsing visit
www.raymondgraceprojects.com

6. *Radionics Rosette (clean)*

See note on p. 178

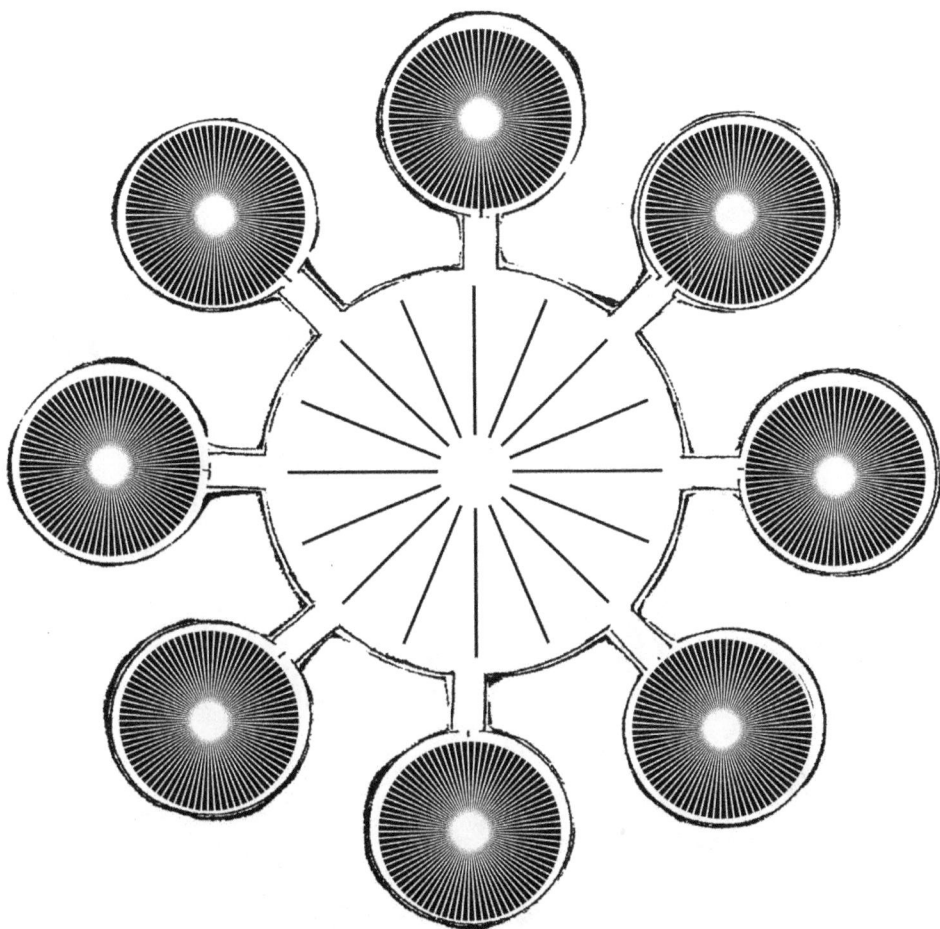

7. Healing Combination No. 4
Back problems

See note on p. 178

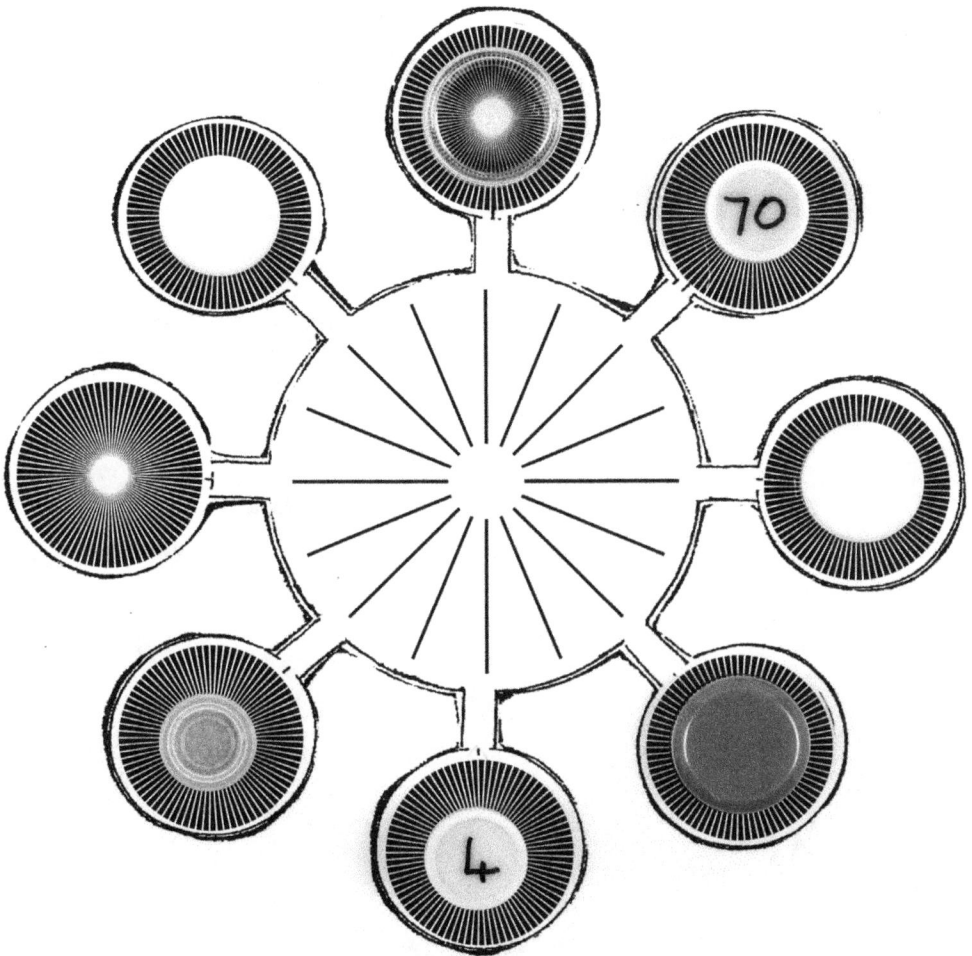

8. Healing Combination No. 10
To increase brain power

See note on p. 178

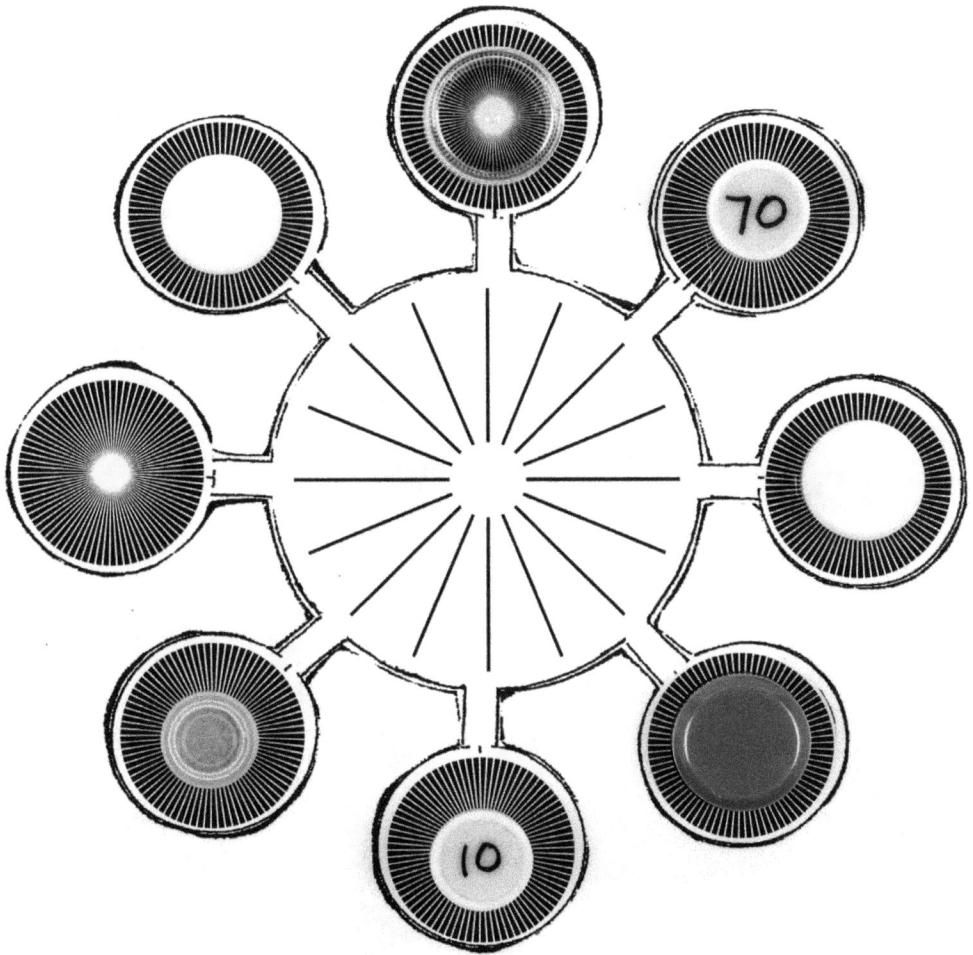

9. Healing Combination No. 12
Kidney Cleanse
See note on p. 178

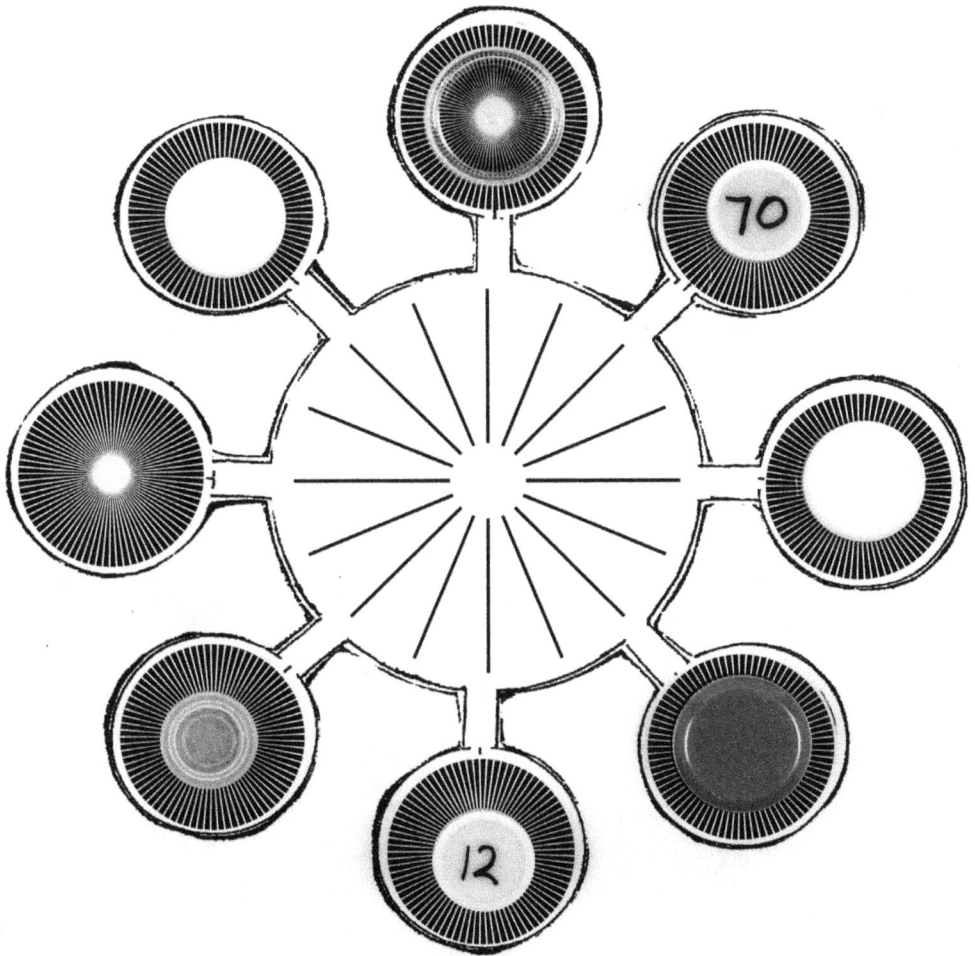

10. Healing Combination No. 15
Diabetes

See note on p. 178

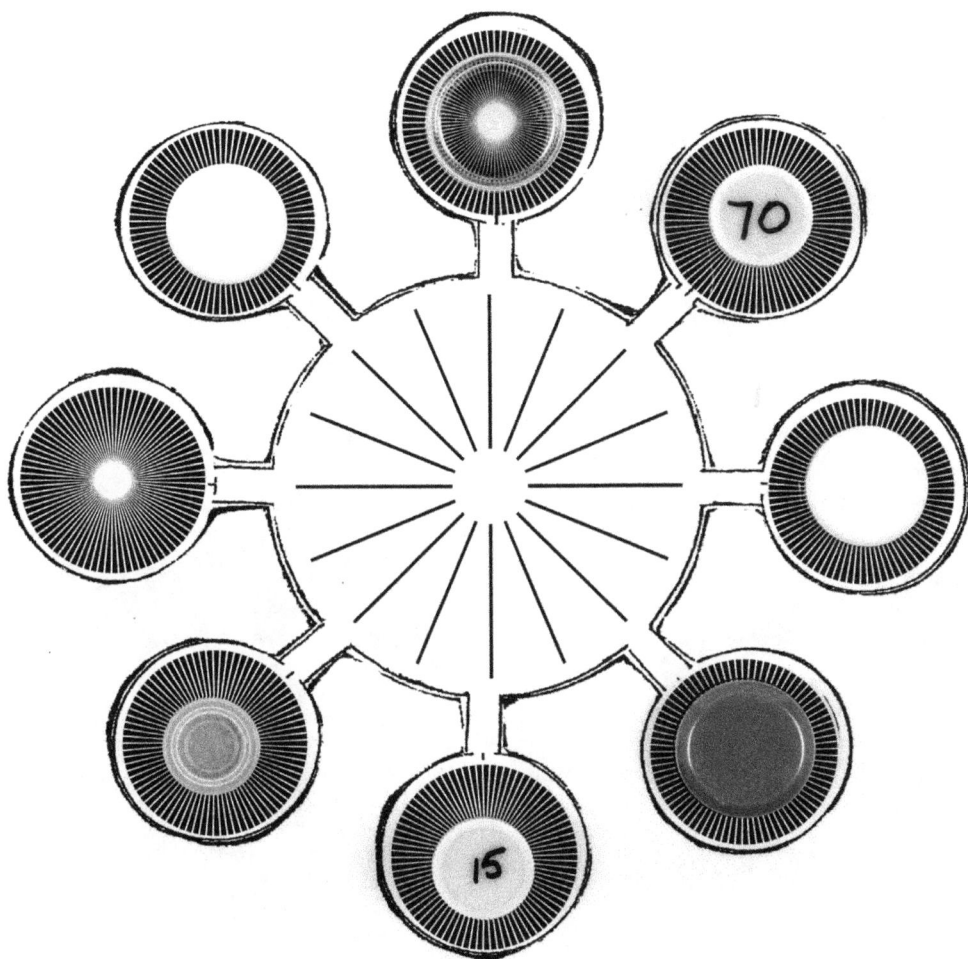

11. Healing Combination No. 24
Headaches

See note on p. 178

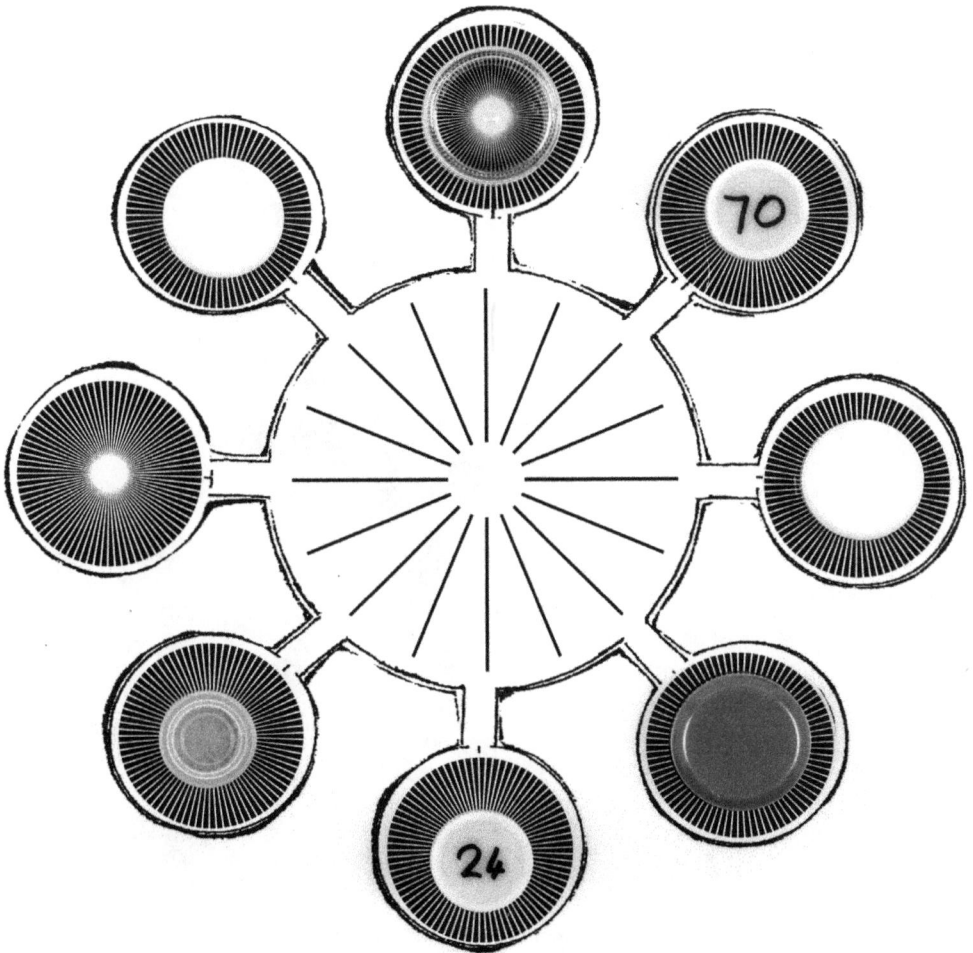

12. Healing Combination No. 25
Heart issues

See note on p. 178

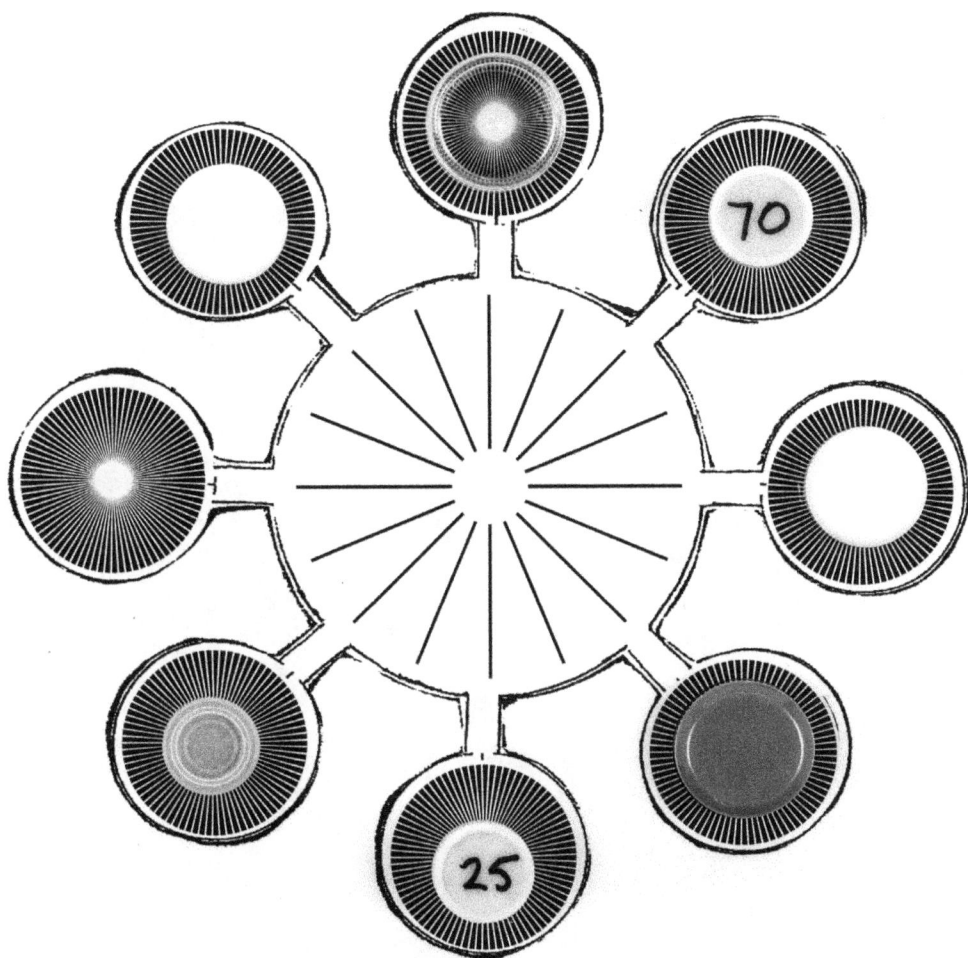

13. Healing Combination No. 27
Liver complaints
See note on p. 178

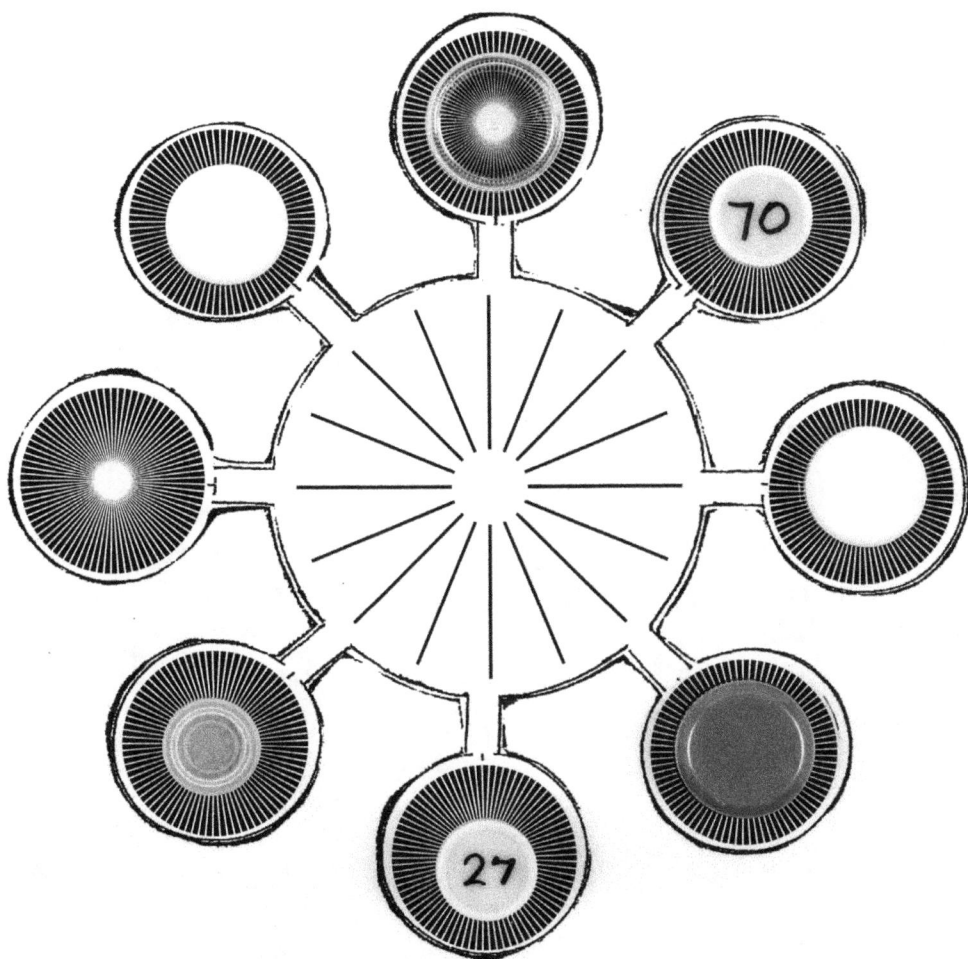

14. Healing Combination No. 31
Infection and inflammation/fever

See note on p. 178

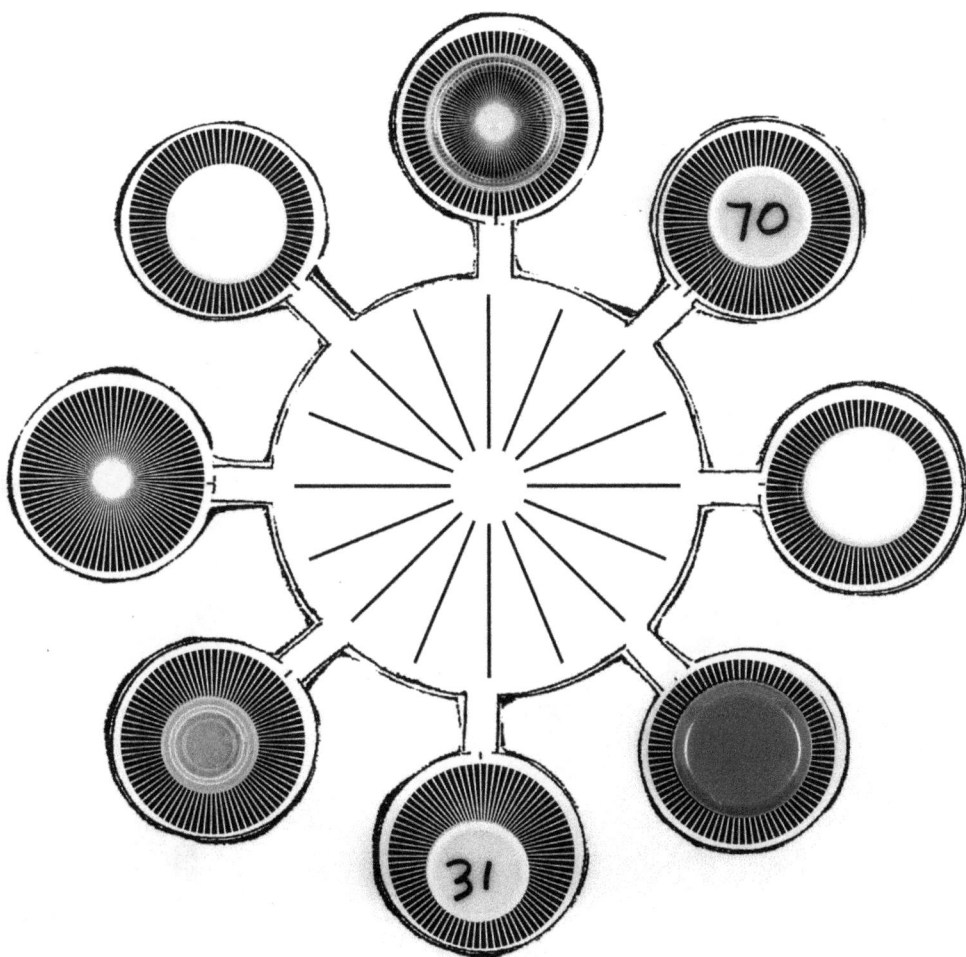

15. Healing Combination No. 40
Addictions

See note on p. 178

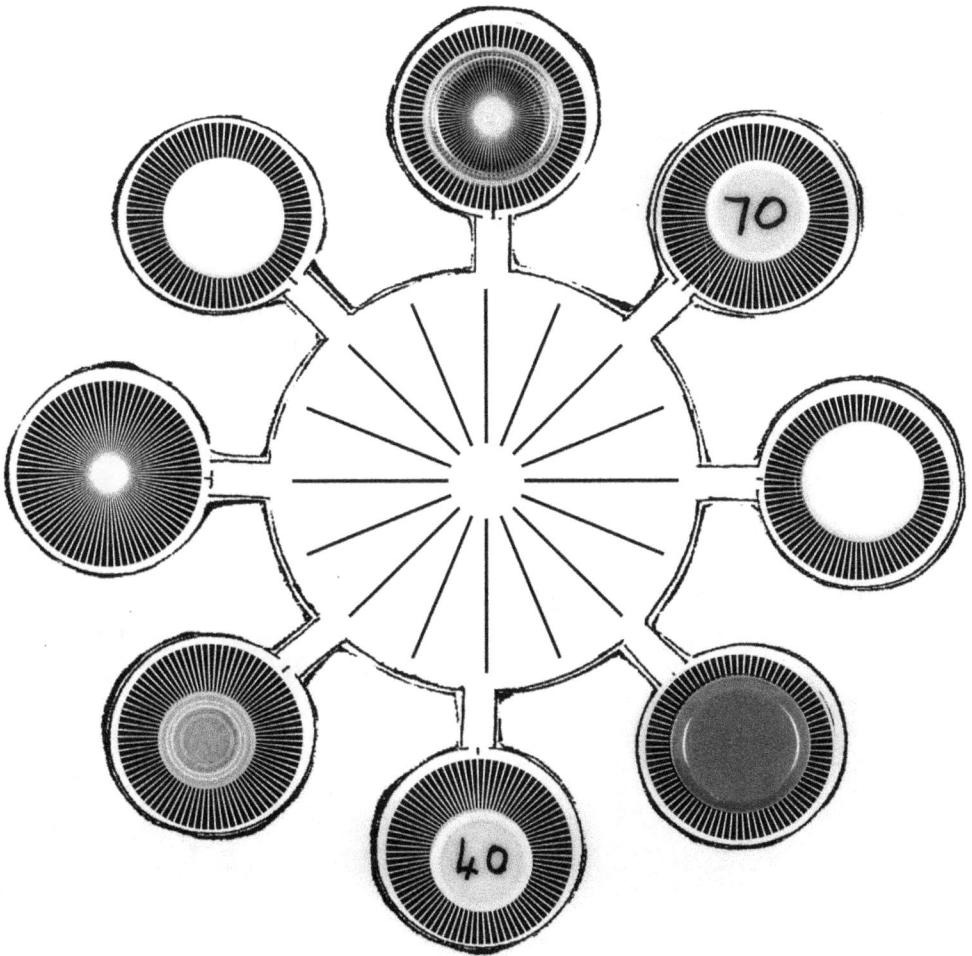

16. Healing Combination No. 59
Removal of negative emotions

See note on p. 178

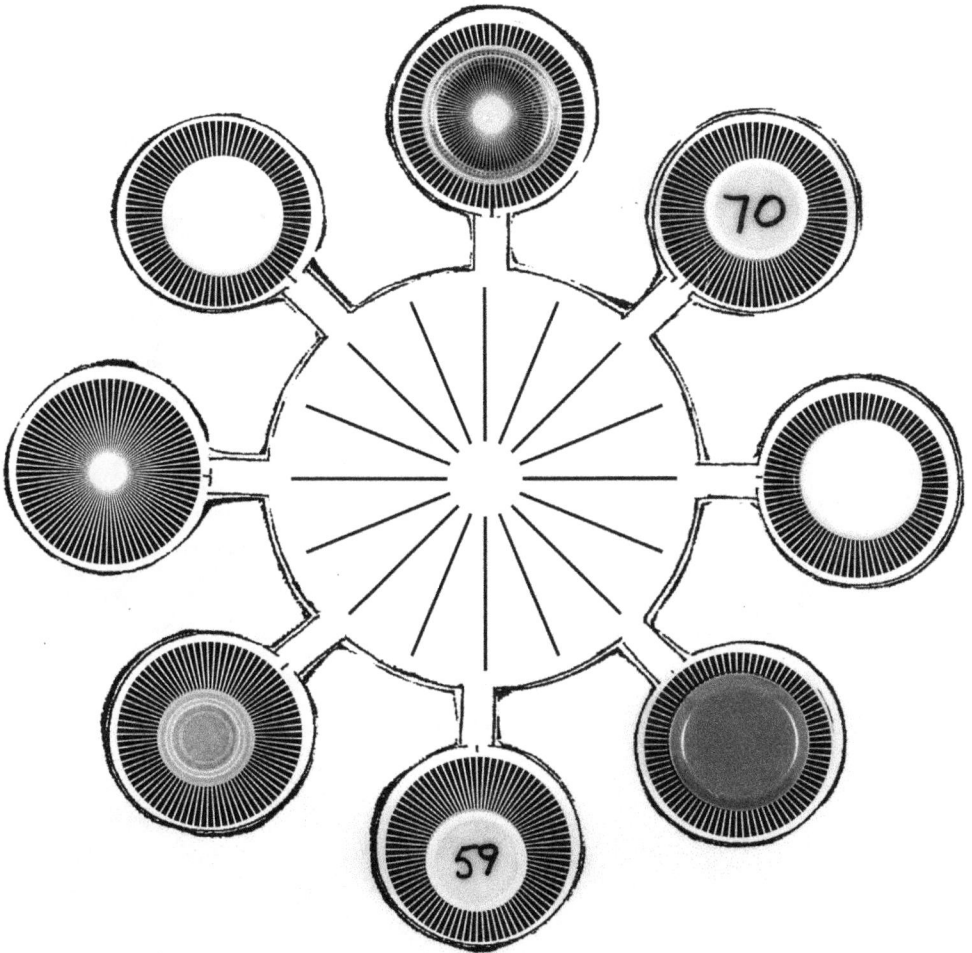

17. Healing Combination No. 70
Total System Tonic (with clearing of toxins)

See note on p. 178

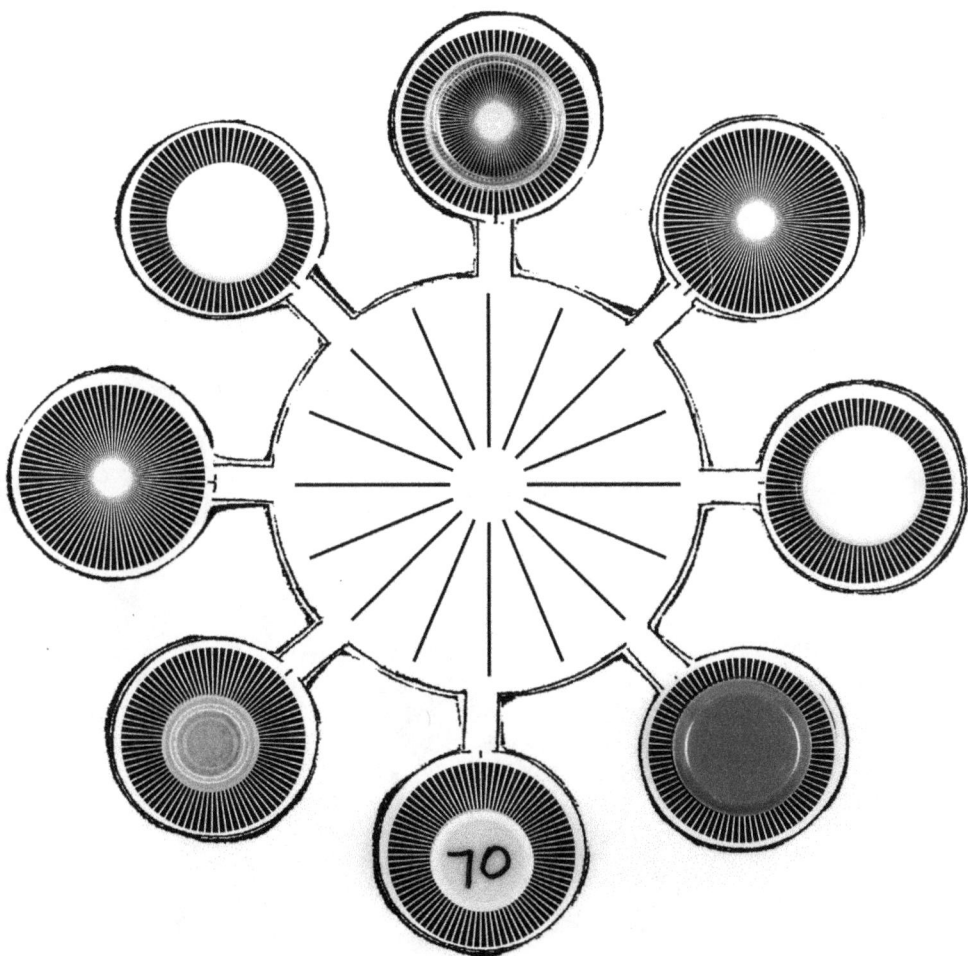

www.ingramcontent.com/pod-product-compliance
Lightning Source LLC
Chambersburg PA
CBHW071547200326
41519CB00021BB/6639